# Contemporary Diagnosis and Management of
# The Enlarged Prostate®

**Kevin T. McVary, MD**
Professor of Urology
Northwestern University
Feinberg School of Medicine
Chicago, IL

**Brian T. Helfand, MD**
Research Assistant Professor of Urology
Northwestern University
Feinberg School of Medicine
Chicago

*First Edition*

Published by Handbooks in Health Care Co.,
Newtown, Pennsylvania, USA

International Standard Book Number: 978-1-931981-77-4

Library of Congress Catalog Card Number: 2007934777

# Table of Contents

This book has been prepared and is presented as a service to the medical community. The information provided reflects the knowledge, experience, and personal opinions of the authors, Kevin T. McVary, MD, Professor of Urology, Northwestern University Feinberg School of Medicine, Chicago, Illinois, and Brian T. Helfand, MD, PhD, Research Assistant Professor of Urology, Northwestern University Feinberg School of Medicine.

**This book is not intended to replace or to be used as a substitute for the complete prescribing information prepared by each manufacturer for each drug. Because of possible variations in drug indications, in dosage information, in newly described toxicities, in drug/drug interactions, and in other items of importance, reference to such complete prescribing information is definitely recommended before any of the drugs discussed are used or prescribed.**

## Chapter 1

# Anatomy of the Prostate Gland

The prostate gland is part of the male reproductive system. Because it wraps around the urethra and enlarges as a man ages, it can cause bothersome urinary symptoms as well as serious health problems in older men.

### Prostate Size and Growth

At birth, the prostate is about the size of a pea.[1] But at puberty, it undergoes rapid, diffuse enlargement under the influence of the male hormone testosterone. By the age of 20, the prostate has reached its normal adult size of 15 to 20 g and is 3 to 4 cm in length.[2] Most men experience a second period of prostate growth in their mid- to late 40s. During those years, the prostate can undergo focal growth in the periurethral region known as the transition zone (TZ), causing the gland to enlarge. Because the enlarged prostate (EP) compresses the urethra, it may obstruct urinary flow (uroflow), which can result in bladder outlet obstruction (BOO) and can lead to lower urinary tract symptoms (LUTS) (Figure 1-1). Prostate gland enlargement affects about 50% of men in their 60s and up to 90% of men in their 70s and 80s.[1]

### Location of the Prostate

The prostate gland is located in the pelvis and lies just below the urinary bladder (Figure 1-2). It is situated

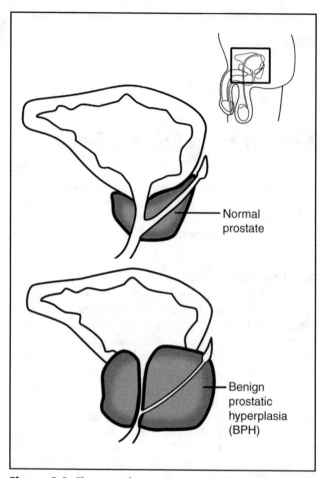

**Figure 1-1:** The normal prostate compared with BPH.

between the pubic bone in front and the rectum behind. The prostate is about the size and shape of a chestnut and wraps around the bladder neck and the proximal end of the urethra (prostatic urethra). Because the prostate is

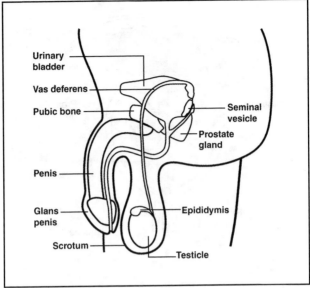

**Figure 1-2:** Location of the prostate gland.

located close to the distal end of the rectum, a digital rectal examination (DRE) is a common method used to assess prostate enlargement and tone.

## Lobes of the Prostate

The prostate gland consists of three lobes: two lateral lobes that are connected anteriorly by an isthmus and posteriorly by a median or middle lobe. The middle lobe lies above and between the ejaculatory ducts, which open into the prostatic urethra to carry semen. The lateral lobes tend to enlarge with age, but the middle lobe is less likely to increase in size.[2] The prostate gland is enclosed in a capsule-like fibromuscular layer. This layer is referred to as the prostatic capsule, although it is not a true capsule because it is an inseparable component of the prostatic stroma.

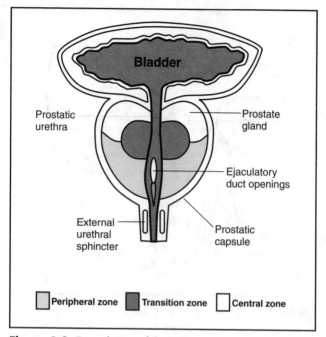

**Figure 1-3:** Frontal view of the normal prostate.

## Prostate Zones

The prostate may be described in terms of three major zones: the TZ, the central zone (CZ), and the peripheral zone (PZ) (Figures 1-3 and 1-4).

### Transition Zone

The TZ is the glandular, innermost part of the prostate, which surrounds the urethra as it passes through the gland. Studies by McNeal[3] demonstrated that nonmalignant proliferation (ie, benign prostatic hyperplasia [BPH]) occurs primarily in the periurethral portion of the TZ. The TZ comprises only about 5% of the glandular prostatic volume and is infrequently the site of prostate cancers (only about 10%).[4]

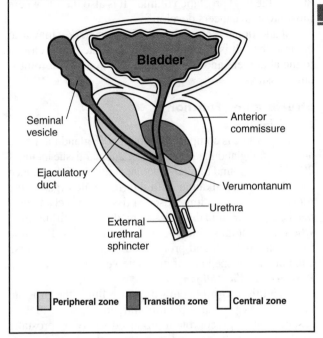

**Figure 1-4:** Sagittal view of the normal prostate.

### Central Zone

The CZ is a nonglandular area that surrounds the TZ. It is composed of dense, stromal tissue that represents approximately 25% of the nonglandular prostatic volume. Like the TZ, it is infrequently the site of malignant prostate cancer growth (about 5% of prostate cancers).[4] The CZ plays an integral role in the development of BPH as it begins to enlarge after the age of 40 and can contribute to difficulties in urination and ejaculation.

### Peripheral Zone

The PZ is located at the back of the prostate gland and is the area closest to the rectum. It comprises approximately

80% of the total prostatic volume.[4] It is also the site where most prostate cancers develop.[2,5]

An additional region, the anterior zone (AZ), may also be described. It is the region of the prostate that is closest to the abdomen, and it is nonglandular, mostly fibromuscular tissue.

## Structure and Function

### Glandular Tissue

The prostate is composed of about 50% glandular tissue and 50% nonglandular tissue.[2] The glandular tissue includes 20 to 30 compound tubular-alveolar acini,[6] which produce a milky, slightly alkaline fluid. During male orgasm, the prostate and surrounding muscular tissue contract and propel the prostatic fluid through several ducts into the urethra, where it combines with sperm from the testes. Prostatic fluid helps nourish and protect sperm during intercourse and constitutes the bulk of ejaculate volume.

### Prostate-specific Antigen

In addition to producing prostatic fluid, the prostate also secretes prostate-specific antigen (PSA), which is an amino-acid glycoprotein produced solely by prostatic epithelial cells. Its production is under the control of circulating androgens that act on androgen receptors.[7] PSA is secreted in the seminal plasma and digests the gel that forms after ejaculation.[7,8] Normally, only small amounts of PSA seep into the circulating androgens, but with prostate disease, PSA levels rise. In addition, prostate massage, ultrasonography, cystoscopic examination, and prostate biopsy can all cause significant elevations in PSA, whereas DRE causes only minimal changes in PSA level.[7]

Although there is an overlap in PSA levels between prostate cancer and BPH, when serum PSA levels are used in conjunction with DRE and/or ultrasonography, it can be a useful diagnostic tool for early detection of cancer. The change in serum PSA levels between two measurements over time (ie, PSA velocity) can also be used to help distinguish between benign prostatic growth and cancer.[9,10] PSA measurements are also useful for monitoring patients after definitive treatment.[7] PSA level is reliable and sensitive in the detection of residual tumors and possibly of recurrence or disease progression after treatment.

### Nonglandular Tissue

Nonglandular tissue of the prostate is fibromuscular stroma.[6] The fibromuscular tissue lies between the glands and contains elastin, collagen, blood vessels, and nerves. The prostate gland has a rich supply of $\alpha$-adrenergic and $\alpha$-cholinergic receptors and nerve fibers, which suggests that the autonomic nervous system may play a role in both the growth and secretory functions of the prostate gland. Nerve complexes referred to as neurovascular bundles are located along the outside of the prostate capsule between the prostate and the rectum. These nerve bundles serve the prostate and are also responsible for erectile function.

## Arterial Supply to the Prostate

### Inferior Vesical Artery

The main arterial blood supply to the prostate gland is from the prostatic branches of the inferior vesical artery (IVA) (Figure 1-5). The IVA commonly originates from the gluteo-pudendal trunk of the internal iliac artery, although it may occasionally branch off from the umbilical artery or the obturator artery.[11] The IVA terminates in capsular and urethral branches that supply the lobes of the prostate. The branches supplying one side of the prostate communicate with the corresponding branches of the other side of the prostate (Figure 1-6).

### Internal Pudendal Artery

The internal pudendal artery (IPA) also originates from the gluteopudendal trunk of the internal iliac artery and provides blood to the prostate, as do small branches of the middle rectal artery (Figure 1-6). One of the terminal branches of the IPA is instrumental in establishing penile erections. It runs through the corpus cavernosum of the

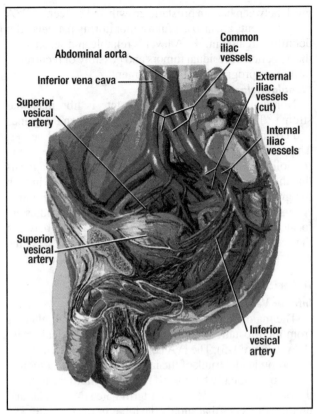

**Figure 1-5:** Arteries and veins of the male pelvis. From Netter FH: *Atlas of Human Anatomy,* 4th ed. Philadephia, PA, Saunders, 2006. Used with permission.

penis and has branches that supply blood to the tissue. The IPA and the corpus cavernosum are the critical vascular structures related to erectile function.[12] Although often difficult to identify, accessory pudendal arteries (APAs) have been observed on the surface of the prostate. These tiny arteries branch off the IPA and may play a role in potency.

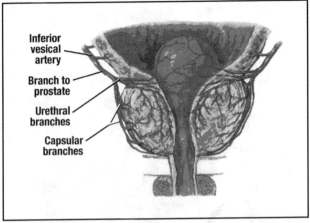

**Figure 1-6:** Arterial supply of the prostate. From Netter FH: *Atlas of Human Anatomy*, 4th ed. Philadephia, PA, Saunders, 2006. Used with permission.

Labels in figure:
- Inferior vesical artery
- Branch to prostate
- Urethral branches
- Capsular branches

For that reason, preservation of the APAs is usually part of the modern radical prostatectomy.[13]

### Atherosclerosis and the Prostate

As a man ages, atherosclerosis may affect blood flow to various parts of the body, including the prostate. Studies by Berger and coworkers[14] and Ghafar and colleagues[15] support the hypothesis that age-related impairment of the blood supply to the prostate has a key role in the development of BPH. Generally considered a progressive disease, BPH is characterized by benign prostatic enlargement (BPE), LUTS, and BOO.

## Nerve Supply to the Prostate

The prostate gland is a richly innervated organ, receiving autonomic innervation from both parasympathetic (cholinergic) and sympathetic (noradrenergic) nerves. Parasympathetic nerves innervate the smooth muscle of the capsule and the space around blood vessels. These

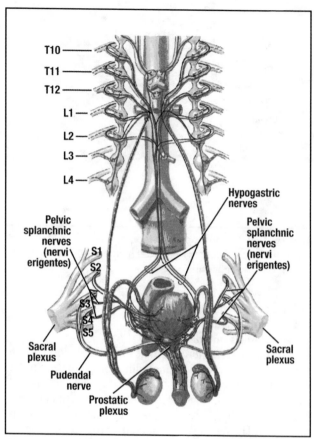

**Figure 1-7:** Innervation of the male reproductive organs. From Netter FH: *Atlas of Human Anatomy,* 4th ed. Philadephia, PA, Saunders, 2006. Used with permission.

nerves are involved in the secretory function of the prostatic epithelium. The sympathetic nerves control prostatic musculature and are responsible for closing the bladder neck during ejaculation.

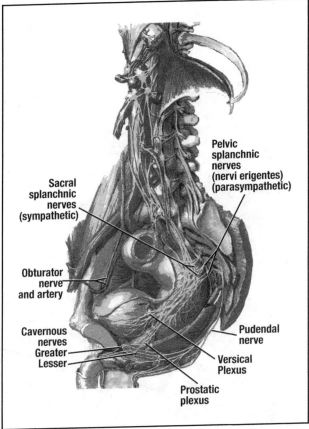

**Figure 1-8:** Nerves of the male pelvic viscera. From Netter FH: *Atlas of Human Anatomy*, 4th ed. Philadephia, PA, Saunders, 2006. Used with permission.

### Pelvic Plexus

The pelvic splanchnic nerves arise from the S2, S3, and S4 sacral roots of the spinal cord. Parasympathetic fibers from these nerves and sympathetic fibers from the hypo-

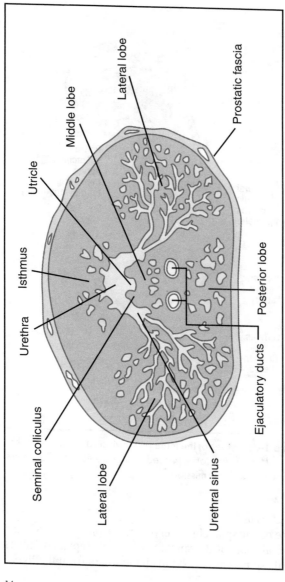

**Figure 1-9:** Cross-section of the prostate. From Netter FH: *Atlas of Human Anatomy*, 4th ed. Philadephia, PA, Saunders, 2006. Used with permission.

gastric nerve (T10-L2) form the pelvic plexus, which is also known as the inferior hypogastric plexus (Figure 1-7).

The pelvic plexus extends into three areas: the anterior section crosses the lateral surface of the seminal vesicles and inferolateral surface of the bladder; the anteroinferior segment runs along the lateral surfaces of the prostate gland; and the inferior section extends between the rectum and the posterolateral surface of the prostate (Figure 1-8). The inferior portion unites with several vessels to form the neurovascular bundle of the prostate.

### Cavernous Nerves

The cavernous nerves originate from the pelvic splanchnic nerves and course along the margin of the pelvic plexus outside the neurovascular bundle. Fibers from the neurovascular bundle innervate the cavernous nerves as well as the prostate, rectum, and levator ani muscles. Fibers from the cavernous nerves innervate the corpus cavernosus, which is vital for an erection. The anatomic location of the cavernous nerves varies, and instead of a single, well-defined trunk, the cavernous nerves are multiple and intertwined with blood vessels and fatty tissue.

## Prostate Anatomy and Ejaculation

Ejaculation is mediated by afferent, efferent, somatic, sympathetic, and parasympathetic fibers through a complex and coordinated sequence of signals.[16] Sperm is produced in the testicles and then travels into the epididymus, where it matures. From the epididymus, the sperm migrates through the two vas deferens tubules, which extend up and around the bladder, and into the seminal vesicles (Figure 1-2).

During the first, or emission, phase of ejaculation, the smooth muscles of the seminal vesicles and the prostate gland contract. Sperm is expelled from the seminal vesicles and travels down through the two ejaculatory ducts and into the prostatic urethra. The ejaculatory ducts pass through the prostate gland on their way to the urethra (Figure 1-9).

Prostatic hyperplasia can compromise the patency of the ejaculatory ducts.

The second or expulsion phase of ejaculation occurs when synchronized relaxation of the external urinary sphincter and concomitant closure of the bladder neck are accompanied by a rhythmic contraction of the striated muscles of the pelvic floor and the bulbospongius muscles.[17] These coordinated processes forcefully expel the semen through the urethra and out the meatus of the penis.

There are four categories of ejaculatory disorders: premature ejaculation, delayed ejaculation, retrograde ejaculation, and anejaculation/anorgasmia.[16] Aging and alterations in the anatomy of the prostate gland have a direct correlation to the presence of ejaculatory dysfunction.[16,18]

## References

1. Men's Health: Prostate gland enlargement. Available at: http://www.mayoclinic.com/health/prostate-gland-enlargement/DS00027. Accessed July 2, 2007.

2. Issa MM, Marshall FF: Anatomy of the genitourinary system. In: *Contemporary Diagnosis and Management of Diseases of the Prostate*, 3rd ed. Newtown, PA, Handbooks in Health Care Co, 2005, pp 5-12.

3. McNeal JE: Origin and evolution of benign prostatic enlargement. *Invest Urol* 1978;15:340-345.

4. Foundation of the Prostate Gland: *Prostate Cancer Treatment Guide*. Available at: http://www.prostate-cancer.com/prostate-cancer-treatment-overview/overview-prostate-anatomy.html. Accessed July 2, 2007.

5. Scher HI: Hyperplastic and malignant diseases of the prostate. In: Braunwald E, Fauci AS, Kasper DL, et al, eds: *Harrison's Principles of Internal Medicine*, 15th ed. New York, NY, McGraw-Hill, 2001, pp 608-616.

6. Marieb EN: The reproductive system. In: *Human Anatomy & Physiology*, 6th ed. San Francisco, CA, Pearson Benjamin Cummings, 2004, pp 1063-1108.

7. el-Shirbiny AM: Prostatic specific antigen. *Adv Clin Chem* 1994; 31:99-133.

8. Stenman UH, Leinonen J, Zhang WM, et al: Prostate-specific antigen. *Semin Cancer Biol* 1999;9:83-93.

9. Loeb S, Catalona WJ: Prostate-specific antigen in clinical practice. *Cancer Lett* 2007;249;30-39.

10. Mochtar CA, Kiemeney LA, Laguna MP, et al: PSA velocity in conservatively managed BPH: can it predict the need for BPH-related invasive therapy? *Prostate* 2006;66:1407-1412.

11. Clegg EJ: The arterial supply of the human prostate and seminal vesicles. *J Anat* 1955;89:209-216.

12. McLaughlin PW, Narayana V, Meirovitz A, et al: Vessel-sparing prostate radiotherapy: dose limitation to critical erectile vascular structures (internal pudendal artery and corpus cavernosum) defined by MRI. *Int J Radiat Oncol Biol Phys* 2005;61:20-31.

13. Secin FP, Touijer K, Mulhall J, et al: Anatomy and preservation of accessory pudendal arteries in laparoscopic radical prostatectomy. *Eur Urol* 2007;51:1229-1235.

14. Berger AP, Bartsch G, Deibl M, et al: Atherosclerosis as a risk factor for benign prostatic hyperplasia. *BJU Int* 2006;98:1038-1042.

15. Ghafar MA, Puchner PJ, Anastasiadis AG, et al: Does the prostatic vascular system contribute to the development of benign prostatic hyperplasia? *Curr Urol Rep* 2002;3:292-296.

16. Wolters JP, Hellstrom WJ: Current concepts in ejaculatory dysfunction. *Rev Urol* 2006;8(8 suppl 4):S18-S25.

17. McMahon CG, Abdo C, Incrocci L: Disorders of orgasm and ejaculation in men. *J Sex Med* 2004;1:58-65.

18. Rosen R, Altwein J, Boyle P, et al: [Lower urinary tract symptoms and male sexual dysfunction: the multinational survey of the aging male (MSAM-7).] *Prog Urol* 2004;14:332-344.

## Chapter 2

# Benign Prostatic Hyperplasia: Natural History, Etiology, and Pathophysiology

Benign prostatic hyperplasia (BPH) remains a confusing and complicated issue for the primary care physician and the urologist. It is a histologic definition related to the stromal and epithelial cell proliferative process, which occurs in the transition zone (TZ) of the prostate.[1,2] This age-related process requires androgens at critical points.[3] Previously, BPH was incorrectly termed benign prostatic hypertrophy, but given the increase in cell numbers that occurs with this growth, hyperplasia, not hypertrophy, is the correct word to use.

Clinical symptoms of BPH occur because of bladder outlet obstruction (BOO) or bladder neck obstruction (BNO) caused by an enlarged prostate (EP) that physically impinges on the prostatic urethra (static component), and by increased smooth muscle tone within the prostatic stroma (dynamic component) (Figure 2-1). Symptomatic or clinical BPH usually refers to the bothersome voiding disturbances known as lower urinary tract symptoms (LUTS) (Table 2-1). LUTS represents a complex of irritative voiding symptoms (ie, nocturia, frequency, urgency) and obstructive voiding symptoms (ie, hesitancy, weak urinary stream, incomplete bladder emptying, straining to

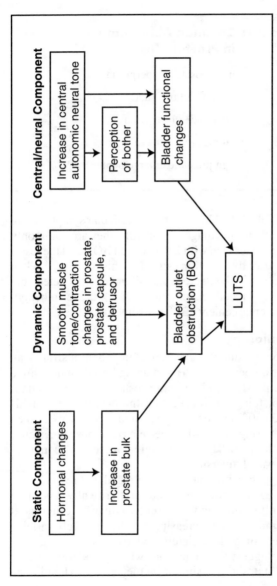

**Figure 2-1:** Diagram depicting the production of lower urinary tract symptoms (LUTS) as a result of increasing activity of the dynamic component and increasing prostatic bulk from enlargement. These components are moderated by variable increases in autonomic neural tone.

## Table 2-1:  Common Abbreviations in Prostate Disease

| | |
|---|---|
| BPH | benign prostatic hyperplasia |
| BOO | bladder outlet obstruction |
| BNO | bladder neck obstruction |
| LUTS | lower urinary tract symptoms |
| BPE | benign prostatic enlargement |

void) (Table 2-2). Although these particular symptoms are not specific for the diagnosis of BPH, they are commonly present in older men with BPH-related BOO and the resultant detrusor dysfunction caused by this process.[1,4] When BPH occurs to the degree that enlargement is detectable upon digital rectal examination (DRE), the term benign prostatic enlargement (BPE) is sometimes used.

## Epidemiology

Autopsy studies have repeatedly demonstrated an association between BPH and aging based on histologic criteria, prostate weight, and prostate volume. Randall[5] found histologic evidence that the occurrence of BPH exceeded 50% in men >50 years and rose to 75% as men entered the eighth decade. Age-related autopsy prevalence of histologic BPH is also similar in several countries despite racial diversity.

Although the literature on the racial and regional impact of BPH is difficult to interpret critically[6,7] because of sampling bias and different evaluation criteria,[8] it clearly indicates an increasing but quantitatively variable incidence of pathologic/clinical BPH with aging. The studies suggest that black and white populations in the United States have a similar incidence of BPH, although

## Table 2-2: Lower Urinary Tract Symptoms

**Irritative**

- Frequency
- Urgency
- Nocturia

**Obstructive**

- Sensation of incomplete bladder emptying
- Decreased or intermittent flow of urinary stream
- Hesitancy
- Straining to void

development of symptoms most likely occurs earlier in black men.[9] Black men in the United States have a higher prevalence of adenomatous hyperplasia than their counterparts on the African continent.

In fact, black men have a significantly higher risk of BPH progression than white men. In a recent study, the efficacy and tolerability of dutasteride (Avodart®) (0.5 mg daily for 2 years) in blacks (n=161), compared with whites (n=3,961), was assessed in a post-hoc analysis of data from three phase 3 clinical trials.[10] Dutasteride significantly reduced serum dihydrotestosterone (DHT) levels by >90% and significantly improved the subjective (ie, International Prostate Symptom Score [IPSS]) and objective (ie, prostate volume, peak urinary flow rate [$Q_{max}$]) risks of BPH-related surgery and acute urinary retention (AUR) outcomes in both blacks and whites. For all efficacy measures, there was no statistically significant treatment-by-race interaction, and dutasteride was well tolerated in both racial groups. The study concluded that dutasteride demonstrated similar efficacy and safety profiles in both blacks and whites.

In April 2007, 5,667 Prostate Cancer Prevention Trial (PCPT) placebo arm participants who were free of BPH at baseline were examined for risk factors associated with symptomatic BPH.[11] The incidence of total BPH was 34.4/1,000 person-years, and it increased 4% ($P<0.001$) with each additional year of age. The trial also revealed that the risk for total BPH was 41% higher in black men ($P<0.03$) and Hispanic men ($P<0.06$) compared with white men, and, for severe BPH, these increases were 68% ($P<0.01$) and 59% ($P<0.03$), respectively. In addition, each 0.05 increase in waist-to-hip ratio (a measure of abdominal obesity) was found to be associated with a 10% increased risk of total ($P<0.003$) and severe ($P<0.02$) BPH. Based on the analysis of the trial data, the researchers concluded that black race, Hispanic ethnicity, and obesity, particularly abdominal obesity, are associated with an increased risk of developing BPH.

Data from the first half of the 20th century indicated a much lower prevalence of BPH in native Chinese and Japanese than in white populations.[8,12] Overall, the data suggest a limited role for race and genetics in the prevalence of histologic BPH, and a larger role for the environment, dietary intake, and genetic factors in the rate and degree of development of BPH that produces a mass.

## Natural History of Benign Prostatic Hyperplasia

Autopsy studies from many countries show the progressive development of BPH with age, starting in some individuals as early as 25 to 30 years.[13] The first pathologic evidence of BPH occurs in <10% of the men in the 31- to 40-year-old group. Evidence of histologic and anatomic BPH increases with age; by the ninth decade, the former is identifiable in approximately 90% and the latter in about >50%.[14] The clinical prevalence of BPH is much lower because it depends on the degree of bothersome symptoms and the patient's ability and desire to seek treatment.

## Table 2-3: Risk Factors for Progression of LUTS

*Histologic prevalence*
- 30% at age 50
- 90% at age 80

*AUA-IPSS >7*
- 12% to 26% at age 40-49
- 46% at age 70+

*Likelihood of treatment*
- 3/1,000 person-years at age 40-49
- 30/1,000 person-years at age 70+

*Progression of disease during 5 years*
- 37% to 42%

*Risk of urinary retention during 1 year*
- 0.3% to 3.5%

*Risk of urinary retention during 5 years*
- 3% to 7%

AUA-IPSS=American Urological Association-International Prostate Symptom Scores

Results from the Olmsted County Study of Urinary Symptoms and Health Status Among Men suggest a measurable progression in symptom severity over 3.5 to 4 years but also suggest that these LUTS may wax and wane over time.[15] The likelihood of progression of LUTS also appears to depend on initial severity of symptoms (Table 2-3). Men with mild urinary symptoms at the beginning of observation (67%) experienced worsened symptoms during a 4-year period (50% progressed to moderate symptoms, 7% to severe symptoms, and 10% chose surgery). Forty-one percent of the men with moderate symptoms at the beginning of observation progressed to severe symptoms, and 24% underwent surgery. Patients with severe symptoms at the initial time of observation (39%) chose surgery during a 4-year period.[16] BPH can lead to complications such as AUR, serious or recurrent urinary tract infections (UTIs), hydronephrosis, bladder calculi, and rarely, renal failure.[15,17-19]

## Etiology

Identifying the etiology of BPH remains a continuing challenge. The universal regional development of histologic BPH in aging men with testes that produce an androgen-diminished environment[20] is an unexplained paradox independent of race and environment. Currently, four hypotheses regarding the etiology of BPH are most prominent: (1) the DHT or altered hormone environment hypothesis; (2) the embryonic reawakening hypothesis; (3) the stem cell hypothesis; and (4) the nonandrogenic testis factor (NATF) hypothesis.[21]

## Pathophysiology

The development and progression of mechanical obstruction from the prostatic mass has been the traditional focus regarding sequelae resulting from BPH. The perception that the mass and configuration of the hyperplasia dictated the degree of outflow blockage undoubtedly resulted from the early experiences in treatment of patients with acute and chronic urinary retention. Renal failure, UTI, and bladder calculi were common indications to relieve BNO. The reversal of these serious secondary phenomena and restoration of improved voiding patterns reinforced the mass concept. Proposals implicating intrinsic prostatic tension from contracting prostate stromal smooth muscle,[22,23] and/or extrinsic tension on the BPH prostate mass by a contracting prostate capsule[24,25] are important to consider in primary or persistent BOO. The role of increased stromal smooth-muscle mediated intrinsic prostate tension has been reinforced by in vitro physiologic and clinical observations with $\alpha$-adrenergic agonists and antagonists (Figure 2-1).[22]

BPH-mediated BOO results in a series of changes in bladder tissue mass, composition, and function. It also affects blood supply and nerve status and function. The degree and persistence of the obstruction are thought to play a pivotal role in the subsequent anatomic and functional bladder effects of BPH. Obstruction can be the primary source of physiologic changes varying from hyperfunction and hyperirritability to nonfunction or atony.

In general, partial bladder obstruction initially results in reversible detrusor hypertrophy and increased bladder weight.[26,27] The increased muscle mass is associated with increased intravesical pressure.[28] Studies in obstructed pigs demonstrate a decrease in functional bladder capacity, increased postvoid residual urine (PVR), detrusor instability associated with incontinence, and a prolonged period of hypoperfusion with associated tissue hypoxia (Figure 2-2).[26]

The anatomic and physiologic alterations that occur in response to obstruction probably play a major role in the specific bladder and renal changes that occur in individual patients. Currently, loss of bladder compliance is most likely the principal factor in producing upper urinary tract functional and anatomic damage. The etiology of obstruction-related involuntary bladder contractions[29] remains elusive, but animal studies suggest they have a myogenic, not neurogenic, basis.[26] Cellules, saccules, and diverticula are related to anatomic bladder changes that have clinical significance and progress unpredictably (Figure 2-2). Based on this experience with the pathophysiology of obstruction-induced bladder changes,[26] BNO should be relieved as soon as possible after diagnosis to maximize the opportunity for bladder recovery.

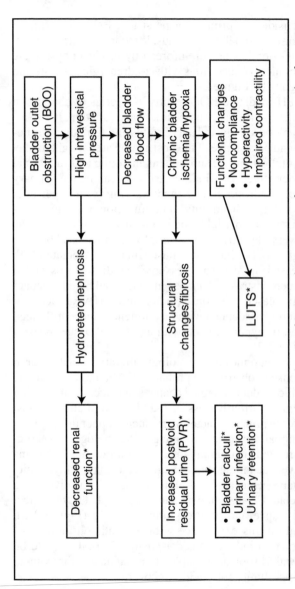

**Figure 2-2:** Diagram depicting the production of LUTS and progression of genitourinary sequelae from BPH. *Denotes pathophysiologic sequelae. LUTS=lower urinary tract symptoms

## Table 2-4: Risk Factors for Erectile Dysfunction (Krimpen Study)*

| Risk Factor | Relative Risk (RR) |
|---|---|
| Age (55-78) | 2.3-14.3 |
| BMI >30 | 3.0 |
| LUTS | 1.8-2.5 |
| Cardiac syndrome | 2.5 |
| COPD | 1.9 |
| Smoking | 1.6 |

*Blanker MH, Bosch JL, Groeneveld FP, et al: Erectile and ejaculatory dysfunction in a community-based sample of men 50 to 78 years old: prevalence, concern, and relation to sexual activity. *Urology* 2001;57:763-768.

BMI=body mass index; COPD=chronic obstructive pulmonary disease; LUTS=lower urinary tract symptoms

## Relationship Between Lower Urinary Tract Symptoms and Erectile Dysfunction

The relationship between LUTS and erectile dysfunction (ED) has received increased attention recently because both diseases are highly prevalent, frequently co-associated in the same aging male group, and contribute significantly to the overall quality of life (QOL) (Table 2-4). The association between these two diseases has also garnered attention as investigators have hypothesized a common pathophysiology to explain the idea that they are causally linked.[30] This common theme hypothesis has taken on a life of its own as pharmaceutical companies have contemplated expanding indications for their drugs for both diseases. The link between ED and LUTS is also important for physicians to understand because the treatment of one disease may adversely affect the other. Almost all accepted therapies for LUTS (surgical or medical) can affect some aspect of sexual health, making it imperative that health-care professionals understand their patients' concerns and motivations in these two linked diseases.

The link between ED and LUTS has biologic plausibility, given the four leading theories of how these diseases interrelate. Each of these explanations has a variable amount of supporting data: (1) nitric oxide (NO) synthase/NO levels decreased or altered in the prostate and penile smooth muscle; (2) autonomic hyperactivity effects on LUTS, prostate growth, and ED; (3) increased Rho-kinase activation activity; and (4) prostate and penile ischemia.[30]

## Relationship Between LUTS and the Metabolic Syndrome

LUTS are a common finding in the aging man. Increasing evidence has recently pointed toward a relationship between LUTS and the metabolic syndrome. This relationship has been supported by recent epidemiologic findings, and possible pathophysiologic links have also been proposed to explain it. The growing prevalence of obesity in the United States makes this link an increasingly relevant problem.

The Third National Health and Nutrition Examination Survey (NHANES III) was a national cross-sectional health survey of 8,814 US men and women conducted between 1988 and 1994.[31] A subset of 2,372 men aged ≥60 years was subsequently evaluated for an association between LUTS and the metabolic syndrome.[30] For this study, LUTS was defined as exhibiting at least three of the following subjective criteria: nocturia, incomplete bladder emptying, weak urinary stream, and urinary hesitancy in men without a history of noncancer prostate surgery.

This study found that the presence of LUTS was strongly associated with an elevated glycosylated hemoglobin $A_{1c}$ ($HbA_{1c}$) level, which is an accurate predictor of a patient's glucose control during the prior 3 months.[32] A history of type 2 diabetes (odds ratio [OR] 1.67) and hypertension (OR 1.76) was also found to correlate with the presence of LUTS. In addition, an inverse association between high-density lipoprotein (HDL) levels and the presence of LUTS was found.[32] An earlier study by the same authors in this patient population also found an association between waist circumference and LUTS. Dahle et al[33] published a case-control study in which abdominal obesity (as measured by the waist-to-hip ratio) and elevated serum insulin levels were significantly associated with an elevated risk of BPH. Further evidence of an epidemiologic link was noted in a study of 943 African-American men between the ages of 40 to 79 years, which found that LUTS was associated with type 2 diabetes, hypertension, and cardiovascular disease.[34] A rising body mass index (BMI) was also found to be a risk factor for the development of BPH in this patient population.[35]

To further evaluate the link between BPH and the metabolic syndrome, 307 men with LUTS were followed by ultrasound to evaluate annual prostate growth rates.[36,37] Several measures of the metabolic syndrome were associated with a greater annual prostate growth rate, including elevated BMI, waist circumference, dyslipidemia, and fasting plasma-insulin levels. Hypertension and noninsulin-dependent type 2 diabetes were also shown to correlate with increased annual rates of prostate growth.[36,37] A correlation between the presence of type 2 diabetes and the increased severity of LUTS was also found in a literature review published in 2001, which surveyed articles on men with concomitant BPH and type 2 diabetes.[38]

Several theoretic pathophysiologic links have been proposed to explain the correlation between the metabolic syndrome and LUTS. Proposed etiologies include changes associated with chronic states of low-grade inflammation, hormonal changes, sympathetic nervous symptom changes, and direct effects of hyperinsulinemia.[39] Elevated blood-glucose levels are a known risk factor for voiding symptoms through osmotic diuresis, which can lead to polyuria and nocturia.[32] Type 2 diabetes can also lead to autonomic neuropathy, which can affect bladder contractility resulting in elevated PVR, weak urinary streams, and voiding frequency.[32] Incomplete bladder emptying combined with glucosuria can also increase the risk of bacterial cystitis, which can contribute to irritative voiding symptoms.

## Summary

The prostate has a unique anatomy and physiology that determines its clinical relevance. This gland is separated into four distinct regions: the peripheral zone (PZ), the central zone (CZ), the TZ, and the periurethral gland region. These zonal variations affect the internal architecture of the prostate as well as its various functions and determine the clinical affect in disease progression. The prostate shows histologic evidence of growth before birth and continues to grow with advancing age. Environmental, dietary intake, and genetic factors appear to play a major role in the development of BPH that produces a mass. There is no consensus as to the exact etiology of the histologic and pathophysiologic process we call BPH. Yet, despite our deficiencies in these aspects, this disease will remain an important topic for physicians and urologists.

## References

1.   Lee C, Kozlowski JM, Grayhack JT: Etiology of benign prostatic hyperplasia. *Urol Clin North Am* 1995;22:237-246.

2.   Lee C, Kozlowski JM, Grayhack JT: Intrinsic and extrinsic factors controlling benign prostatic growth. *Prostate* 1997;31:131-138.

3.   Partin AW, Oesterling JE, Epstein JI, et al: Influence of age and endocrine factors on the volume of benign prostatic hyperplasia. *J Urol* 1991;145:405-409.

4.   Bruskewitz R: Management of symptomatic BPH in the US: who is treated and how? *Eur Urol* 1999;36(suppl 3):7-13.

5.   Randall A: *Surgical Pathology of Prostatic Obstruction.* Baltimore, MD, Williams & Wilkins Co, 1931.

6.   Lytton B, Emery JM, Harvard BM: The incidence of benign prostatic obstruction. *J Urol* 1968;99:639-645.

7.   Ekman P: BPH epidemiology and risk factors. *Prostate Suppl* 1989;2:23-31.

8.   Oishi K, Boyle P, Barry MJ, et al: Epidemiology and natural history of benign prostatic hyperplasia. In: Denis L, Griffiths K, Khoury S, et al, eds: *Fourth International Consultation on BPH Proceedings.* Health Publications, Plymouth, England, 1998, pp 23-59.

9.   Derbes VD, Leche SM, Hooker CC: The incidence of benign prostatic hypertrophy among the whites and negroes of New Orleans. *J Urol* 1937;38:383.

10.   Roehrborn CG, Ray P: Efficacy and tolerability of the dual $5\alpha$-reductase inhibitor, dutasteride, in the treatment of benign prostatic hyperplasia in African-American men. *Prostate Cancer Prostatic Dis* 2006;9:432-438.

11.   Kristal AR, Arnold KB, Schenk JM, et al: Race/ethnicity, obesity, health related behaviors and the risk of symptomatic benign prostatic hyperplasia: results from the prostate cancer prevention trial. *J Urol* 2007;177:1395-1400.

12.   Rotkin ID: Origins, distribution and risk of benign prostatic hypertrophy. In: Hinman F Jr, ed: *Benign Prostatic Hypertrophy.* New York, NY, Springer-Verlag, 1983, pp 10-21.

13.   McNeal JE, Redwine EA, Freiha FS, et al: Zonal distribution of prostatic adenocarcinoma. Correlation with histologic pattern and direction of spread. *Am J Surg Pathol* 1988;12:897-906.

14.   Harbitz TB, Haugen OA: Histology of the prostate in elderly men. A study in an autopsy series. *Acta Pathol Microbiol Scand [A]* 1972;80:756-768.

15.   McPherson K, Wennberg JE, Hovind OB, et al: Small-area variations in the use of common surgical procedures: an interna-

tional comparison of New England, England, and Norway. *N Engl J Med* 1982;307:1310-1314.

16. Guess HA, Jacobsen SJ, Girman CJ, et al: The role of community-based longitudinal studies in evaluating treatment effects. Example: benign prostatic hyperplasia. *Med Care* 1995;33(4 suppl): AS26-AS35.

17. Di Silverio F, Gentile V, Pastore AL, et al: Benign prostatic hyperplasia: what about a campaign for prevention? *Urol Int* 2004;72:179-188.

18. O'Leary MP: Lower urinary tract symptoms/benign prostatic hyperplasia: maintaining symptom control and reducing complications. *Urology* 2003;62(3 suppl 1):15-23.

19. Jacobsen SJ, Girman CJ, Guess HA, et al: Natural history of prostatism: longitudinal changes in voiding symptoms in community dwelling men. *J Urol* 1996;155:595-600.

20. Gray A, Feldman HA, McKinlay JB, et al: Age, disease, and changing sex hormone levels in middle-aged men: results of the Massachusetts Male Aging Study. *J Clin Endocrinol Metab* 1991;73:1016-1025.

21. Grayhack JT, Sensibar JA, Ilio KY, et al: Synergistic action of steroids and spermatocele fluid on in vitro proliferation of prostate stroma. *J Urol* 1998;159:2202-2209.

22. Caine M, Pfau A, Perlberg S: The use of alpha-adrenergic blockers in benign prostatic obstruction. *Br J Urol* 1976;48:255-263.

23. Lepor H: Adrenergic blockers for the treatment of benign prostatic hyperplasia in prostatic diseases. In: Lepor H, ed: *Prostatic Diseases*. WB Saunders Co, Philadelphia, PA, 2000, pp 297-307.

24. Hutch JA, Rambo OS, Jr: A study of the anatomy of the prostate, prostatic urethra and the urinary sphincter system. *J Urol* 1970;104:443-452.

25. Ohnishi K: [A study of the physical properties of the prostate (second report)—the relationships between dysuria and the strength of the surgical capsule in benign prostatic hypertrophy]. *Nippon Hinyokika Gakkai Zasshi* 1986;77:1388-1399.

26. McConnell JD: Bladder responses to obstruction. In: Kirby R, McConnell J, Fitzpatrick J, et al, eds: *Textbook of Benign Prostatic*

*Hyperplasia*. Oxford, England, ISIS Medical Media Ltd, 1996, pp 105-108.

27. Levin RM, Brading AF, Mills IW, et al: Experimental models of bladder outlet obstruction in prostatic disease. In: Lepor H, ed: *Prostatic Diseases*. WB Saunders Co, Philadelphia, PA, 2000, pp 169-196.

28. Claridge M, Shuttleworth KE: The dynamics of obstructed micturition. *Invest Urol* 1964;2:188-199.

29. Schoenberg HW, Gutrich JM, Cote R: Urodynamics studies in benign prostatic hypertrophy. *Urology* 1979;14:634-637.

30. McVary KT: Erectile dysfunction and lower urinary tract symptoms secondary to BPH. *Eur Urol* 2005;47:838-845.

31. Ford ES, Giles WH, Dietz WH: Prevalence of the metabolic syndrome among US adults: findings from the third National Health and Nutrition Examination Survey. *JAMA* 2002;287:356-359.

32. Rohrmann S, Smit E, Giovannucci E, et al: Association between markers of the metabolic syndrome and lower urinary tract symptoms in the Third National Health and Nutrition Examination Survey (NHANES III). *Int J Obes (Lond)* 2005;29:310-316.

33. Dahle SE, Chokkalingam AP, Gao YT, et al: Body size and serum levels of insulin and leptin in relation to the risk of benign prostatic hyperplasia. *J Urol* 2002;168:599-604.

34. Joseph MA, Harlow SD, Wei JT, et al: Risk factors for lower urinary tract symptoms in a population-based sample of African-American men. *Am J Epidemiol* 2003;157:906-914.

35. Joseph MA, Wei JT, Harlow SD, et al: Relationship of serum sex-steroid hormones and prostate volume in African American men. *Prostate* 2002;53:322-329.

36. Hammarsten J, Hogstedt B: Clinical, anthropometric, metabolic and insulin profile of men with fast annual growth rates of benign prostatic hyperplasia. *Blood Press* 1999;8:29-36.

37. Hammarsten J, Hogstedt B: Hyperinsulinaemia as a risk factor for developing benign prostatic hyperplasia. *Eur Urol* 2001;39:151-158.

38. Boon TA, Van Venrooij GE, Eckhardt MD: Effect of diabetes mellitus on lower urinary tract symptoms and dysfunction in

patients with benign prostatic hyperplasia. *Curr Urol Rep* 2001;2: 297-301.

39. Kasturi S, Russell S, McVary KT: Metabolic syndrome and lower urinary tract symptoms secondary to benign prostatic hyperplasia. *Curr Urol Rep* 2006;7:288-292.

# Chapter 3

# Diagnoses

A patient usually seeks treatment for lower urinary tract symptoms (LUTS) when benign prostatic hyperplasia (BPH) obstructs his urine outflow, sometimes painfully, and impairs the quality of his life (ie, sense of bother). When patients present to a health-care provider, a history should be taken and an evaluation made based on both a physical examination and testing. All men who have LUTS due to BPH should receive at least a yearly examination to monitor the progression of symptoms.

## History

An initial history should exclude other causes of the obstructed urinary flow (uroflow) and include an inquiry about hematuria and previous urinary tract problems. Neurologic disorders (eg, diabetes mellitus, stroke, Parkinson's disease) can similarly impair bladder function, as can prostatitis, urinary tract infection (UTI), neoplasms of the bladder or prostate, urethral stricture or injury, and neurogenic bladder. A review of the patient's medications will determine whether those medications can diminish bladder contractility (ie, anticholinergics [antihistamines]) or increase outflow resistance (ie, sympathomimetics [decongestants]).

An index developed by the American Urological Association (AUA) allows for proven reliable scoring of BPH symptoms as well as response to treatment, the AUA Symptom Index (AUA-SI) (Table 3-1). This index does not diagnose

## Table 3-1: AUA-SI for BPH*

**For Questions 1–6, circle the number associated with the answer that best describes your symptom:**

1. Over the past month, how often have you had a sensation of not emptying your bladder completely after urinating?

2. Over the past month, how often have you had to urinate again less than 2 hours after you finished urinating?

3. Over the past month, how often have you found you stopped and started again several times while urinating?

4. Over the past month, how often have you found it difficult to postpone urination?

5. Over the past month, how often have you had a weak stream while urinating?

6. Over the past month, how often have you had to push or strain to begin urinating?

**For Question 7, circle the number associated with the answer that best describes your symptoms:**

7. Over the past month, how many times did you typically get up to urinate from the time you went to bed until the time you got up in the morning?

TOTAL OF ALL CIRCLED ANSWERS IN QUESTIONS 1-7: ___

*Barry MJ, Fowler FJ, O'Leary MP, et al: The American Urological Association symptom index for benign prostatic hyperplasia. The Measurement Committee of the American Urological Association. *J Urol* 1992;148:1549-1557; discussion 1564.

| Not At All | < 1 Time in 5 | < 1/2 The Time | ~1/2 The Time | > 1/2 The Time | Almost Always |
|---|---|---|---|---|---|
| 0 | 1 | 2 | 3 | 4 | 5 |
| 0 | 1 | 2 | 3 | 4 | 5 |
| 0 | 1 | 2 | 3 | 4 | 5 |
| 0 | 1 | 2 | 3 | 4 | 5 |
| 0 | 1 | 2 | 3 | 4 | 5 |
| 0 | 1 | 2 | 3 | 4 | 5 |

| None | One Time | Two Times | Three Times | Four Times | Five or More Times |
|---|---|---|---|---|---|
| 0 | 1 | 2 | 3 | 4 | 5 |

## Table 3-2: BPH Impact Index[*]

Instructions: For each question, check the one box that best describes your urinary condition.

1. Over the past month, how much physical discomfort did any urinary problems cause you?

   $\square_0$ none  $\square_1$ only a little  $\square_2$ some  $\square_3$ a lot

2. Over the past month, how much did you worry about your health because of any urinary problems?

   $\square_0$ none  $\square_1$ only a little  $\square_2$ some  $\square_3$ a lot

3. Overall, how bothersome has any trouble with urination been during the past month?

   $\square_0$ not at all bothersome  $\square_1$ bothers me a little little  $\square_2$ bothers me some  $\square_3$ bothers me a lot

4. Over the past month, how much of the time has any urinary problem kept you from doing the kinds of things you would usually do?

   $\square_0$ none of the time  $\square_1$ a little of the time  $\square_2$ some of the time  $\square_3$ most of the time  $\square_4$ all of the time

[*]Fowler FJ, Barry MJ: Quality of life assessment for evaluating benign prostatic hyperplasia treatments. An example of using a condition-specific index. *Eur Urol* 1993;24(suppl 1):24-27.

LUTS; it grades its severity. The self-administered test can be used to help assess BPH symptom severity. A score of 0 to 7 indicates mild symptoms; 8 to 19, moderate symptoms; and 20 to 35, severe symptoms. Patients should be asked to fill out the questionnaire at the time of initial presentation, following various treatments and before any invasive treatment (ie, before surgery). Because LUTS can sometimes be present without bother, it is important to assess the patient's sense of bother from LUTS by using the BPH Impact Index (B II) (Table 3-2). Additionally, because alterations in sexual function accompany LUTS (either preceding it or as a result of a LUTS due to BPH treatment), some quantitative assessment of sexual function domains should be considered (Table 3-3). Patients will also sometimes report concurrent sexual dysfunction; therefore, questions addressing erectile, ejaculatory, and libido function should also be asked (Table 3-4). The use of these indices is meant to augment a detailed history, not replace it.

## Physical Examination

A digital rectal examination (DRE) of the prostate and an assessment of anal sphincter tone help estimate the size of the prostate gland as well as uncover other potential LUTS causes. Where the normal prostate is rounded, heart-shaped, and about the size of a chestnut, an affected gland will feel symmetrically enlarged, smooth, and firm, though slightly elastic; and will seem to protrude into the rectal lumen. Significant findings of induration, nodularity, or asymmetry should be further investigated for the possibility of prostate cancer. The examination should also include a lower extremity assessment for edema, peripheral pulses, and neurologic reflexes. Lower extremity edema may indicate the presence of LUTS related to the mobilization of third spaced fluid upon recumbancy rather than bladder outlet obstruction (BOO). A focused neurologic examination of lower extremity and saddle regions may reveal occult neurologic causes of LUTS. Bladder palpation may also detect retention.

## Testing

Tests to consider include urinalysis, renal ultrasonography, uroflowmetry, postvoid residual urine (PVR) volume measurement, and transrectal ultrasonography (TRUS)

## Table 3-3: International Index of Erectile Function[*]

**Instructions:** For each question, check the one box that best describes your condition.

*In the past month/week:*

1. How often were you able to get an erection during sexual activity?

   - $\square_0$ no sexual activity
   - $\square_1$ never or almost never
   - $\square_2$ a few times (much less than half the time)
   - $\square_3$ sometimes (about half the time)
   - $\square_4$ most times (much more than half the time)
   - $\square_5$ always or almost always

2. When you had erections with sexual stimulation, how often were your erections hard enough for penetration?

   - $\square_0$ no sexual activity
   - $\square_1$ never or almost never
   - $\square_2$ a few times (much less than half the time)
   - $\square_3$ sometimes (about half the time)
   - $\square_4$ most times (much more than half the time)
   - $\square_5$ always or almost always

[*]Rosen RC, Riley A, Wagner G, et al: The international index of erectile function (IIEF): a multidimensional scale for assessment of erectile dysfunction. *Urology* 1997;49:822-830.

3. When you attempted sexual intercourse, how often were you able to penetrate (enter) your partner?

- $\square_0$ did not attempt sexual intercourse
- $\square_1$ never or almost never
- $\square_2$ a few times (much less than half the time)
- $\square_3$ sometimes (about half the time)
- $\square_4$ most times (much more than half the time)
- $\square_5$ always or almost always

4. During sexual intercourse, how often were you able to maintain your erection after you had penetrated (entered) your partner?

- $\square_0$ did not attempt sexual intercourse
- $\square_1$ never or almost never
- $\square_2$ a few times (much less than half the time)
- $\square_3$ sometimes (about half the time)
- $\square_4$ most times (much more than half the time)
- $\square_5$ always or almost always

*continued on next page*

## Table 3-3: International Index of Erectile Function*
### (continued)

5. During sexual intercourse, how difficult was it to maintain your erection to completion of intercourse?

☐ 0 did not attempt intercourse
☐ 1 extremely difficult
☐ 2 very difficult
☐ 3 difficult
☐ 4 slightly difficult
☐ 5 not difficult

6. How do you rate your confidence that you could get and keep an erection?

☐ 1 very low
☐ 2 low
☐ 3 moderate
☐ 4 high
☐ 5 very high

7. When you had sexual stimulation or intercourse, how often did you ejaculate?

☐ 0 no sexual stimulation or intercourse
☐ 1 never or almost never
☐ 2 a few times (much less than half the time)
☐ 3 sometimes (about half the time)
☐ 4 most times (much more than half the time)
☐ 5 always or almost always

*Rosen RC, Riley A, Wagner G, et al: The international index of erectile function (IIEF): a multidimensional scale for assessment of erectile dysfunction. *Urology* 1997;49:822-830.

8. When you had sexual stimulation or intercourse, how often did you have the feeling of orgasm or climax?

- [ ] $_0$ no sexual stimulation or intercourse
- [ ] $_1$ never or almost never
- [ ] $_2$ a few times (much less than half the time)
- [ ] $_3$ sometimes (about half the time)
- [ ] $_4$ most times (much more than half the time)
- [ ] $_5$ always or almost always

9. If you had to spend the rest of your life with your erectile condition just the way it is now, how would you feel about that?

- [ ] $_1$ very dissatisfied
- [ ] $_2$ moderately dissatisfied
- [ ] $_3$ about equally satisfied and dissatisfied
- [ ] $_4$ moderately satisfied
- [ ] $_5$ very satisfied

3

## Table 3-4: Male Sexual Health Questionnaire to Assess Ejaculatory Dysfunction[*]

*In the past month:*
**Ejaculatory Function[**]**

| 1. How often have you been able to ejaculate or cum when having sexual activity? | All of the time (5) | Most of the time (4) |
| --- | --- | --- |
| 2. How would you rate the strength or force of your ejaculation? | As strong as it always was (5) | A little less strong than it used to be (4) |
| 3. How would you rate the amount or volume of semen or fluid when you ejaculate? | As much as it always was (5) | A little less than it used to be (4) |

**Bother/Satisfaction[***]**

| 4. If you have had any ejaculation difficulties or have been unable to ejaculate, have you been bothered by this? | No problem with ejaculation (0) | Not at all bothered (1) |
| --- | --- | --- |

[*]Rosen RC, et al: Development and validation of a four-item version of the male sexual health questionnaire to assess ejaculatory dysfunction (MSHQ-EjD short form). *Urology* 2007;69:805-809.

[**]The ejaculatory function score, which is the sum of the ordinal responses to the three items, can range from 1 to 15.

[***]The bother/satisfaction score can range from 0 to 5.

| About half of the time (3) | Less than half of the time (2) | None of the time /Could not ejaculate (1) | |
|---|---|---|---|
| Somewhat less strong than it used to be (3) | Much less strong than it used to be (2) | Very much less strong than it used to be (1) | Could not ejaculate (0) |
| Somewhat less than it used to be (3) | Much less than it used to be (2) | Very much less than it used to be (1) | Could not ejaculate (0) |

| A little bothered (2) | Moderately bothered (3) | Very bothered (4) | Extremely bothered (5) |
|---|---|---|---|

in conjunction with a biopsy for those men with elevated prostate-specific antigen (PSA) levels. TRUS alone is rarely indicated unless prostatic abscess is suspected or unless treatment decisions are to be based on total prostatic volume (ie, use of combination therapy [see below] or transurethral resection of the prostate [TURP] vs open simple prostatectomy). TRUS will help assess prostate size, which can be important in selected patients in whom prostate size may determine the need for additional treatment. However, the routine use of TRUS should be avoided. Although TRUS and magnetic resonance imaging (MRI) are limited by their high cost and availability, they are the most accurate methods of estimating prostate volume. In contrast, DRE is inexpensive but notoriously underestimates prostatic volume. It is recommended that if knowing the size of the prostate is crucial for patient care, then the patient should undergo either TRUS (or MRI) to accurately determine prostate volume.

The following tests should be considered when a patient presents with bothersome LUTS:

- A urinalysis will indicate blood, marked glycosuria (consider unrecognized diabetes mellitus), marked proteinuria (consider nephritis), or an infection in the urine. This is a mandatory test for every patient with LUTS.
- Serum PSA is a recommended part of the evaluation in men with LUTS. A serum PSA test is used as a screening tool for prostate cancer as well as a potential proxy for prostate volume. This can be a useful tool in deciding the use of adding medications that reduce prostate volume and affect the risk for progression. Elevated serum PSA has been shown to correlate with the progression of BPH.[1,2] PSA is produced almost exclusively by the epithelial cells of the prostate. Increased levels of serum PSA are present in patients with increased prostate volume (ie, BPH, prostate cancer). Elevated serum PSA in patients with BPH has also been shown to be associated with a higher incidence of surgical treatments and acute urinary

retention (AUR).[3] In addition, elevated serum PSA levels at the initial evaluation for BPH have been associated with increased bothersome LUTS, faster symptom deterioration, reduced uroflow rate, and an impaired quality of life (QOL). Therefore, serum PSA values >1.3 ng/mL are associated with increased BPH progression.[3,4]

- A serum creatinine level test is recommended only when the health-care provider suspects upper urinary tract deterioration, increased PVR volumes, or another disease that can affect overall renal function.

- For those patients with a history of urinary tract surgery, an elevated serum creatinine level, hematuria, UTI, or renal calculi, a renal ultrasonography or another imaging test will help to evaluate the risk of recurrence or residual after-effect as the cause. A renal ultrasonography is not a recommended routine test.

- A uroflowmetry test may support the presence of BPH symptoms by demonstrating a reduced peak urinary flow rate ($Q_{max}$) and prolonged flow time. Use of the flow rate has been questioned because it does not assess bladder contractility and cannot rule out alternative causes of LUTS. However, measuring the uroflow rate can be useful in assessing treatment response (Table 3-1). A uroflow rate >15 mL/sec is normal or signifies only mild disease, 10 to 15 mL/sec is often associated with moderate symptoms, and <10 mL/sec can indicate severe BPH. At extremely low voided volumes (ie, <150 mL), uroflow results are inaccurate, and results from such voiding episodes should be viewed with a high degree of skepticism.[5] Furthermore, it must be remembered that normal flow-rate parameters vary with voided volume and age. The progressive decrease in $Q_{max}$ observed with age does not appear to be the result of an increased incidence of BOO.[6,7] A variety of nomograms with volume- and/or age-adjusted normative flow-rate calculations has been published. The Siroky nomogram is one of the most commonly used (Figure 3-1A and 3-1B).[8,9]

**Figure 3-1A and 3-1B:** Siroky nomogram for evaluation of urinary flow (uroflow) results. The peak urinary flow rate ($Q_{max}$) (vertical axis) and total bladder volume (voided volume plus residual volume, horizontal axis) are plotted as a single point on the nomogram. The shaded zone indicates values that occur in <2.5% of the normal male population. Siroky nomogram facilitates comparison of average flow rates (Figure 3-1A) and $Q_{max}$ (Figure 3-1B) regardless of volume voided. $Q_{max}$ varies with volume voided. It is generally accepted that voided volumes of <150 mL generate inaccurate flow patterns.

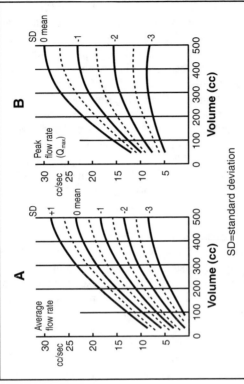

SD=standard deviation

The Siroky nomograms are designed to allow the comparison of flow rates regardless of volume. By consensus, the use of uroflowmetry cannot differentiate between outflow obstruction and impaired contractility. From Siroky MB, Olsson CA, Krane RJ: *J Urol* 1979;122:665-668.

- Increased volume of PVR, another indicator of BPH, can be measured by either catheterization or ultrasound. The ultrasound method, which is less invasive, is more commonly used, but less accurate.
- Urine cytology can be a useful diagnostic test when the practitioner is concerned about the possibility of bladder carcinoma mimicking LUTS due to BPH. A urine cytology test should not be done routinely.
- Cystoscopy is an elective procedure in the evaluation of LUTS due to BPH. Reasons for considering this somewhat invasive diagnostic examination include concerns about the etiology of the underlying BOO (urethral stricture vs benign prostatic enlargement [BPE]) or if a predominance of irritative complaints makes one wonder if bladder cancer is present.

A voiding diary is a useful and inexpensive means to assess if fluid-drinking behavior or other lifestyle issues are complicating the presentation of LUTS. A voiding diary is particularly helpful in those patients who complain about nocturia. To create a voiding diary, a patient records the time, the concomitant activity, and the type of fluid and volume of his urine over three consecutive 24-hour periods. The patient is simultaneously asked to record the time, volume, and type of activity undertaken during each void in the same 3-day period. These diary entries should be reviewed with the patient during his next office visit to see if any behavior changes can be instituted to lessen LUTS.

## Advanced Urodynamics and the Evaluation of LUTS

The purpose of urodynamic testing is to reproduce the patient's symptoms in a controlled laboratory setting and to demonstrate the putative cause of the voiding complaint. Pressure-flow studies are advantageous because they can be used to differentiate detrusor hypocontractility from BOO, and are considered the 'gold standard' for the diagnosis of BOO. However, pressure-flow testing is invasive, time consuming, labor intensive, and prone to measurement error. Two or three consecutive studies must be performed because the results of a single test are highly variable.[10] Reasons to perform urodynamic studies in men with LUTS generally fall into two categories—absolute and relative indications. The absolute indications include failure of previous surgery, known or suspected neurologic disease, prior pelvic radiation, and prior radical pelvic surgery. The relative indications include severe symptoms and normal uroflow results, young age, and isolated symptoms of urgency and urge incontinence.

## Pressure-Flow Studies

Pressure-flow studies consist of the simultaneous measurement of bladder pressure, abdominal pressure, and uroflow. The patient presents with a full bladder, and a free (uncatheterized) uroflow rate will be obtained. A small (7-8F) dual lumen catheter is placed in each urethra; one lumen is used to measure bladder pressure and the other is used to infuse room-temperature water or saline. A rectal catheter is placed to measure abdominal pressure. Detrusor pressure (pdet) is obtained by subtracting abdominal pressure from total bladder pressure. Electromyography (EMG) of the external urethral sphincter also is usually recorded via patch or needle electrodes on the perineum. The bladder is filled through the urethral catheter at a medium rate (10 to 50 mL/min). When the patient's bladder feels full, he is asked to void. A high pdet/low flow pattern indicates BOO, while a low pdet/low flow pattern indicates impaired detrusor contractility. The EMG recording indicates the degree of external sphincter activity and is most useful in identifying a lack of sphincter relaxation during voiding (ie, dynamic obstruction).

There are a variety of ways in which the results of pressure-flow studies may be interpreted. In general, a pdet of >40 cm $H_2O$ with a uroflow <12 mL is considered obstructed, a pdet of <30 cm $H_2O$ with a uroflow <12 mL

## Table 3-5: Uroflowmetry—Interpretation of Peak Urinary Flow Rate

| $Q_{max}$ | Explanation |
| --- | --- |
| >15 mL/s | Normal or mild disease only |
| 10-15 mL/s | Moderate obstruction/symptoms |
| <10 mL/s | Severe obstruction/symptoms |

$Q_{max}$=peak urinary flow rate

## Table 3-6: Interpretation of Pressure-Flow Studies

| Pdet at Maximum Flow | $Q_{max}$ | Explanation |
| --- | --- | --- |
| >40 mm Hg | <12 mL/s | Obstructed |
| 30-40 mm Hg | <12mL/s | Indeterminate |
| <30 mm Hg | <12 mL/s | Impaired detrusor contractility |

$Q_{max}$=peak urinary flow rate

indicates impaired detrusor contractility, and a pdet between 30 and 40 cm $H_2O$ with a uroflow <12 mL is indeterminate (Table 3-5).[11] Another way to analyze pressure-flow studies is to plot the pdet at maximum flow vs $Q_{max}$ (Table 3-6). The Abrams-Griffiths nomogram is then used to group results into obstructed, unobstructed, and equivocal categories (Figure 3-2).

There tends to be a decrease in obstructive parameters with successive pressure-flow studies, so that as many as 28% of patients will be redefined into a less obstructive Abrams-Griffiths category if the first study is compared

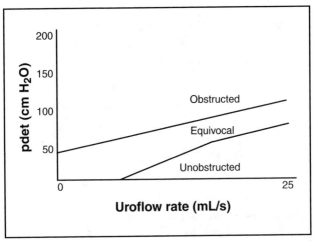

**Figure 3-2:** Abrams-Griffith nomogram for evaluation of pressure-flow data in men. Detrusor pressure (pdet) at peak flow (vertical axis) and $Q_{max}$ (horizontal axis) are plotted as a single point. More sophisticated analyses may be performed to attempt to classify patients whose results are in the equivocal area. The Abrams-Griffiths nomogram is used to divide results into obstructed, unobstructed, and equivocal categories using the values obtained from the simultaneous measurement of bladder pressure and urinary flow (uroflow) rate throughout the micturition cycle. The x-axis represents $Q_{max}$, while the y-axis represents the pdet at the moment that $Q_{max}$ is reached.

with subsequent studies. Furthermore, interpretation of these tests is not always straightforward, resulting in a high intra- and inter-interpreter variability.[12]

## Videourodynamics

Videourodynamic studies involve the measurement of urodynamic parameters, along with the simultaneous fluoroscopic imaging of the bladder and urethra. For these studies, contrast material is infused into the bladder instead of saline or water. The term videourodynamics may be used to describe a number of different techniques. In some instances, fluoroscopy is simply added to a pressure-flow study, as described above. In other cases, a triple-lumen bladder catheter is used, with the third, proximal lumen used to measure intraluminal urethral pressure. During filling, the proximal urethral pressure transducer (which is marked with a radio-opaque marker) is positioned at the area of maximum resting urethral pressure (the external sphincter), while the distal transducer remains in the bladder to record intravesical pressure. This technique gives a more direct measurement of external sphincter activity than EMG electrodes.

By adding fluoroscopic imaging to the measurements of pressures and flow rates, videourodynamic testing can identify the location of BOO (eg, bladder neck, prostate, external urethral sphincter, bulbar urethra). Furthermore, other abnormalities, such as vesicoureteral reflux or urinary incontinence, are easily discovered.

No urodynamic criteria have currently been found that predict treatment response to medical treatment for men with LUTS. Therefore, urodynamic testing has a limited role before the initiation of medical treatment. The role of routine urodynamic testing before surgery is controversial. Urodynamic testing does appear to lower the surgical failure rate. Furthermore, despite the fact that a significant number of unobstructed patients benefit from surgery, it is unclear what is being treated. Alternative therapies, such as anticholinergic agents or biofeedback-assisted pelvic floor muscle exercises, may be equally beneficial and less morbid. The decision to obtain urodynamic studies must be individualized for each patient, but the eventual decision is usually based on the treatment philosophy of the physician.

A decision tree for evaluating a patient for BPH would follow a logical path (Figure 3-3). Upon detection of LUTS, an initial evaluation would determine the need to start BPH

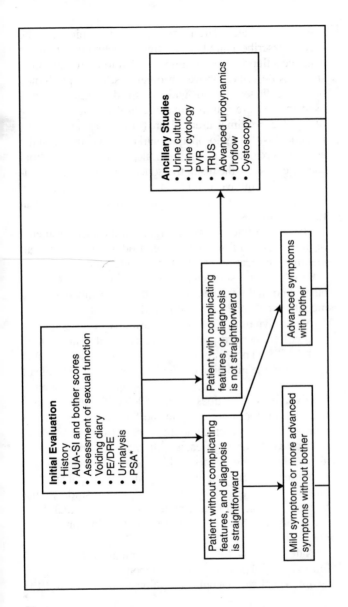

**Initial Evaluation**
- History
- AUA-SI and bother scores
- Assessment of sexual function
- Voiding diary
- PE/DRE
- Urinalysis
- PSA*

Patient without complicating features, and diagnosis is straightforward

Patient with complicating features, or diagnosis is not straightforward

Mild symptoms or more advanced symptoms without bother

Advanced symptoms with bother

**Ancillary Studies**
- Urine culture
- Urine cytology
- PVR
- TRUS
- Advanced urodynamics
- Uroflow
- Cystoscopy

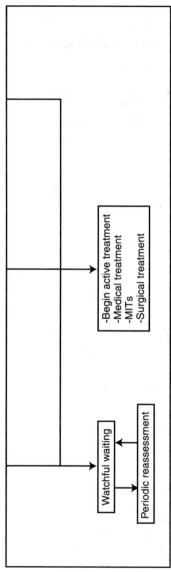

**Figure 3-3:** Algorithm for the initial assessment and diagnosis of lower urinary tract symptoms (LUTS) due to benign prostatic hyperplasia (BPH).

AUA=American Urological Association; AUA-SI=American Urological Association Symptom Index; DRE=digital rectal examination; MITs=minimally invasive treatments; PE=prostate enlargement; PSA=prostate-specific antigen; PVR=postvoid residual urine; TRUS=transrectal ultrasonography

* In men with a life expectancy of >10 years in whom the diagnosis of prostate cancer can alter LUTS due to BPH management.

Watchful waiting

Periodic reassessment

Begin active treatment
-Medical treatment
-MITs
-Surgical treatment

### Table 3-7: Comparing BPH, Prostate Cancer, and Prostatitis

| | BPH |
|---|---|
| **Findings on DRE** | Symmetrically enlarged, rubbery, nontender gland |
| **PSA levels** | Elevations tend to mirror increases in gland size |
| **TRUS** | Homogeneous appearance with regular borders |
| **Biopsy** | Hyperplasia present |
| **Systemic symptoms** | None usually |
| **Onset of LUTS** | Gradual |
| **Prostatic fluid** | No bacteria |

BPH=benign prostatic hyperplasia; DRE=digital rectal examination; LUTS=lower urinary tract symptoms; PSA=prostate-specific antigen; TRUS=transrectal ultrasonography

treatment or continue testing to eliminate the possibility of other similar symptomatic disorders.

Abnormal findings would include PSA levels above age-appropriate norms, increased PSA velocity (>75 ng/dL/year), or >4 ng/dL indicating the need for a repeat PSA test or biopsy. Other potential causes of LUTS to screen for include bacterial infections with accompanying inflammation, nonbacterial inflammation (nonbacterial prostatitis), and prostate cancer. Because the treatment for each of these conditions is different, a correct diagno-

| Prostate Cancer | Prostatitis |
| --- | --- |
| Asymmetric gland with hardened areas | Enlarged, tender gland |
| Elevations even without PE; faster increases over time | |
| Tumors with irregular margins | |
| Cancer cells present | |
| | Fever, chills, malaise |
| | Rapid |
| | Bacteria present |

sis is imperative. Key differences that help differentiate BPH from prostate cancer and prostatitis are summarized in Table 3-7.

## References

1. Anderson JB, Roehrborn CG, Schalken JA, et al: The progression of benign prostatic hyperplasia: examining the evidence and determining the risk. *Eur Urol* 2001;39:390-399.

2. Partin AW: Etiology of Benign Prostatic Hyperplasia. In: Lepor H, ed: *Prostatic Diseases.* Philadelphia, PA, WB Saunders Co, 2000, pp 95-105.

3.   Isaacs JT, Coffey DS: Changes in dihydrotestosterone metabolism associated with the development of canine benign prostatic hyperplasia. *Endocrinology* 1981;108:445-453.

4.   McConnell JD, Akakura K, Bartsch G, et al: Hormonal treatment of benign prostatic hyperplasia. In: Cockett ATK, Khoury S, Aso Y, eds: *The 2nd International Consultation on Benign Prostatic Hyperplasia (BPH), Proceedings 2*. Paris, France, Scientific Communication International, 1993, p 417.

5.   Drach GW, Layton TN, Binard WJ: Male peak urinary flow rate: relationships to volume voided and age. *J Urol* 1979;122:210-214.

6.   Girman CJ, Panser LA, Chute CG, et al: Natural history of prostatism: urinary flow rates in a community-based study. *J Urol* 1993;150:887-892.

7.   Madersbacher S, Klingler HC, Schatzl G, et al: Age related urodynamic changes in patients with benign prostatic hyperplasia. *J Urol* 1996;156:1662-1667.

8.   Siroky MB, Olsson CA, Krane RJ: The flow rate nomogram: I. Development. *J Urol* 1979;122:665-668.

9.   Siroky MB, Olsson CA, Krane RJ: The flow rate nomogram: II. Clinical correlation. *J Urol* 1980;123:208-210.

10.  Sonke GS, Kortmann BB, Verbeek AL, et al: Variability of pressure-flow studies in men with lower urinary tract symptoms. *Neurourol Urodyn* 2000;19:637-651; discussion 651-666.

11.  Blaivas JG: Obstructive uropathy in the male. *Urol Clin North Am* 1996;23:373-384.

12.  Kortmann BB, Sonke GS, Wijkstra H, et al: Intra- and inter-investigator variation in the analysis of pressure-flow studies in men with lower urinary tract symptoms. *Neurourol Urodyn* 2000; 19:221-232.

## Chapter 4

# Medical Therapy

C hoosing the correct therapy options for patients who present with urinary symptoms related to benign prostatic hyperplasia (BPH) can be a complicated issue. As previously mentioned, BPH is a histologic diagnosis that refers to the proliferation of smooth muscle and epithelial cells within the transition zone (TZ) of the prostate.[1,2] The clinical manifestations of BPH occur because the enlarged prostate (EP) physically obstructs the bladder outlet (static component, ie, the mechanical and physical compression exerted upon the prostatic urethra by the increased mass of an EP), as well as causes increasing smooth muscle tone and resistance (dynamic component, ie, increased prostatic smooth muscle tone caused by smooth muscle cell proliferation and increased neural input).[3]

The treatment interventions for clinical BPH have been traditionally directed toward the alleviation of bothersome lower urinary tract symptoms (LUTS). However, within the past several years, there has also been an interest in treating BPH to prevent associated comorbidities (eg, acute urinary retention [AUR], renal insufficiency, detrusor dysfunction, development of bladder calculi, progressive worsening of LUTS, urinary incontinence, and recurrent urinary tract infection [UTI]).[4,5] The mainstay treatment options for BPH have changed dramatically over the past decades, evolving from a paradigm that relied almost exclusively

## Table 4-1: Types of Medical Therapies for BPH

- Hormonal therapy
- 5α-Reductase inhibitors (5ARIs)
- α-Adrenergic antagonists
- Combination therapy
- Phytotherapy

on surgery to one focused on medical therapy.[6] Recent US Medicare data have shown that the number of prostatectomies for BPH-related disease has decreased from 250,000 in the mid-1980s to 88,000 in 1997.[7,8] This decrease in the number of prostatectomies, in lieu of the increasing number of men diagnosed with clinical BPH each year, is likely multifactoral. However, the most apparent reason is the development of safe, effective medical therapies. This chapter will focus on the medical therapies available for the treatment of symptomatic BPH. There are currently a number of different types of medical therapies available, as outlined in Table 4-1.

## Hormonal Therapy

To date, the mechanisms or molecular pathways associated with the histologic development of BPH have not been elucidated. However, current beliefs assert that BPH is a multifactorial process involving interactions between prostatic cells, the endocrine system, neural influences, heredity, and environmental factors.[9] Of these factors, one of the most important is the effect of testicular androgens on prostate cell growth. Therefore, the regulation of testicular hormone function is integral to the medical therapy of BPH.

It has been demonstrated that adequate levels of circulating testosterone are necessary for normal prostatic development and growth. This is essential during early development, but also appears to be the major driving factor for prostate enlargement (PE) in BPH. The hypothalamic/adrenal/gonadal axis plays an integral part in regulating testosterone levels; gonadotropin-releasing hormone (GnRH) is released in a pulsatile fashion by the hypothalamus of the brain into the portal-venous circulation, stimulating the anterior pituitary to secrete luteinizing hormone (LH). LH enters the systemic circulation, stimulating the Leydig cells of the testes to release testosterone (Figure 4-1). In addition, testicular androgens are also simultaneously being released from the adrenal gland. For this process to occur, the hypothalamus releases corticotropin-releasing hormone (CRH) that acts upon the anterior pituitary gland and stimulates the release of corticotropins. Corticotropins then act upon cells within the zona fasciculata and zona reticulata of the adrenal gland, inducing the release of androgens, such as dehydroepiandrosterone sulfate. Of circulating androgens, 95% are released from the testes and the remaining 5% are released from the adrenal glands. Approximately 98% of circulating androgens are bound to plasma proteins, such as albumin and sex hormone-binding globulin (SHBG).[10] Only free testosterone is biologically active and available to enter prostate cells by a simple diffusion process.

However, before testosterone can exert its effects on the prostatic cells, it has to undergo a modification to become dihydrotestosterone (DHT). Testosterone is converted to its active metabolite DHT by the enzyme $5\alpha$-reductase. DHT forms a complex with androgen receptors, which is then transported to the nucleus. Within the nucleus, this complex exerts its effects on the transcription of DNA. These effects are necessary for the development of the prostate gland, as well as the normal growth and hyperplasia of the prostate.

Drugs, such as finasteride (Proscar®) and dutasteride (Avodart®), have been developed to specifically target and

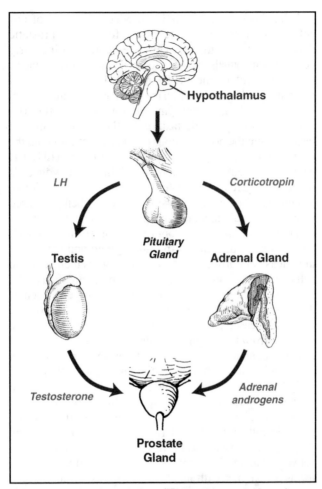

**Figure 4-1:** The hypothalamic/adrenal/gonadal axis for androgen production. The hypothalamus stimulates the pituitary to release luteinizing hormone (LH), which then stimulates Leydig cells in the testes to produce testosterone. In a similar fashion, the hypothalamus also signals the pituitary to release corticotropin, which stimulates androgen production within the adrenal gland.

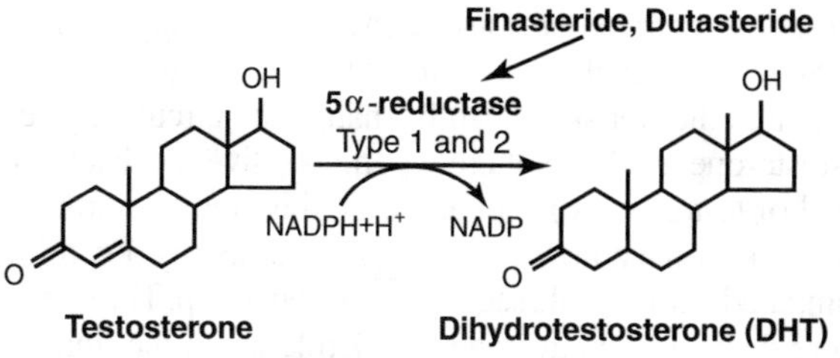

**Figure 4-2:** The mechanism of action of 5ARIs. There are two isozymes of 5α-reductase, types 1 and 2. The type 1 isozyme is expressed mainly in the skin, whereas the type 2 isozyme is expressed in the prostate, seminal vesicles, and epidiymis. Within cells, testosterone is modified by either type 1 or type 2 5α-reductase to form dihydrotestosterone (DHT). DHT is responsible for gene activation, which stimulates cellular growth and division. Therefore, inhibitors of this enzyme, such as finasteride (Proscar®) and dutasteride (Avodart®), prevent prostatic growth and thus have efficacy in the treatment of BPH. While dutasteride inhibits both isozymes, its side-effect profile and efficacy are similar to finasteride.

inhibit the enzyme 5α-reductase (Figure 4-2). These drugs virtually eliminate the production of DHT, thus inhibiting normal prostate growth and hyperplasia. For example, finasteride administration results in an 80% to 90% decrease in the concentration of DHT within both the prostate and the general circulation, while dutasteride decreases DHT >90%.[11,12] Accompanying this response is a 56% increase in the local concentration of testosterone within the prostate, without a significant change in the total serum concentration of testosterone.[13-15]

### Finasteride

Finasteride is a 5α-reductase inhibitor (5ARI) that exerts its effects on the prostate gland by inhibiting the formation of DHT (Figure 4-2). The first study to report the efficacy of finasteride was a 1-year multicenter, randomized, double-blind, placebo-controlled clinical trial. The data obtained from the study demonstrated a mean decrease in circulating DHT levels by 80%. This level was sustained for the 12 months of treatment and did not significantly change the circulating serum testosterone levels (ie, there was no positive feedback on the level of testosterone).[16] In addition, this study demonstrated the peak urinary flow rate ($Q_{max}$) increased by 1.6 mL/sec, compared with 0.2 mL/sec in the placebo group. The symptom score decreased an average of 2.7 mL/sec in the finasteride group compared with 1 mL/sec in the placebo group.

The Proscar Long-Term Efficacy and Safety Study (PLESS) trial continues to be the largest clinical study to investigate the effects of finasteride on the management of BPH.[17] In this multicenter, double-blind, placebo-controlled study conducted in the United States, more than 3,000 men with moderate-to-severe LUTS and an EP on digital rectal examination (DRE) were randomized to a finasteride group (5 mg/day) or a placebo group. During the 4-year study period, 10% of the 1,516 men in the placebo group and only 5% of the 1,524 men in the finasteride group underwent surgery for BPH (a 55% reduction in risk with the use of finasteride). AUR developed in about 7% of the men in the placebo group and about 3% of the men in the finasteride group (a 57% reduction in risk with the use of finasteride). There was a significant ($P$ <0.001) decrease in the mean American Urological Association-International Prostate Symptom Scores (AUA-IPSS), with a 3.3-point reduction in the finasteride group and a 1.3-point reduction in the placebo group. Treatment with finasteride improved urinary flow (uroflow) rates and significantly ($P$ <0.001) reduced prostate volume. This study suggested that long-term medical therapy could affect the natural history of BPH as manifested by AUR and surgery. A 5ARI is now recommended as prevention for BPH because it may alter the condition's natural history. In addition, this class of medications is recommended for patients with large prostates (>30 g) and moderate-to-severe symptoms of BPH.

Prostate cancer is the most common cancer affecting men and the third most common cause of cancer death in American men. Early detection of prostate cancer has been enhanced by the introduction of the serum prostate-specific antigen (PSA) screening assay.[18] PSA is an enzyme produced by the prostate gland and is detectable at low levels in the blood in patients who do not have cancer or inflammation. Most men with prostate cancer have elevated serum PSA levels. In addition, PSA levels rise (albeit quite slowly) as prostate volume increases due to BPH.[19,20]

Treatment with finasteride decreases serum PSA levels by about 50% over a 4- to 6-month period.[21-23] Because BPH and prostate cancer can co-exist in the same patient, there has been concern as to the ability to detect prostate cancer in patients taking 5ARIs. Stoner[24] demonstrated that despite about a 60% decrease in intraprostatic concentrations of testosterone, there appears to be no increased risk of prostate cancer for patients taking finasteride. Doubling the serum PSA for patients taking finasteride and then interpreting the resulting PSA value in untreated men has been recommended.[23] Oesterling et al[25] suggested that mathematically doubling the serum PSA level approximates it and permits adequate interpretation of PSA for cancer detection in finasteride-treated patients. Any sustained increases in PSA levels during finasteride treatment should be carefully evaluated with a prostate biopsy. To date, 5ARIs have been shown to play a role in the reduction of PSA levels in the incidence of prostate cancer. However, it should be noted that a recent report demonstrated a significant increase in more aggressive prostate cancer types in those patients who were diagnosed with prostate cancer after taking a 5ARI.[26,27]

### Dutasteride

Because it is responsible for the production of DHT, the enzyme 5α-reductase occurs as two different isozymes, known as type 1 and type 2. The prostate gland predominantly expresses the type 2 isozyme, while the skin and liver express an abundance of the type 1 isozyme.[28-30] The contribution of DHT is primarily derived from the type 2 isozyme found in the prostate stromal tissue. However, type 1 5α-reductase in the liver, skin, and a small amount in the prostate may play a role in prostate enlargement (PE).

Dutasteride, a drug developed for the treatment of BPH, is a dual inhibitor of both the type 1 and type 2 5α-reductase isozymes.[31] Like finasteride, dutasteride has been shown to significantly suppress DHT levels (>90%), thus decreasing LUTS due to BPH.[32,33] In addition, it has been shown to significantly decrease prostate volume (about 50%), increase uroflow rate (about 30%), decrease the risk of AUR, and decrease the risk of requiring BPH-related surgery compared with placebo.[32] By decreasing prostate size, dutasteride is also useful in the prevention of BPH progression.[34]

### Other Hormone Manipulations for the Treatment of BPH

Inhibiting both testosterone and DHT production prevents the formation of BPH. Castration is a way to inhibit the production of these hormones and can be achieved by chemical means. For example, androgen-receptor antagonists, such as flutamide, progestin/estrogen combinations, and GnRH agonists, have been used to decrease androgen levels and treat patients with BPH. The data demonstrate that these drugs can be quite effective in reducing prostate size and improving symptoms.[35] However, their cost and relatively increased frequency of adverse effects (ie, decreased libido, painful gynecomastia, hot flashes) have excluded these drugs from routine clinical use.

It has been demonstrated that estrogens exert effects upon the prostate gland and contribute to the pathophysiology of BPH. As men age, there is a direct correlation between prostate volume and increased serum levels of estradiol and estriol.[36] In a canine model of BPH, experiments have shown that estrogens act synergistically with androgens to promote BPH. The hormones increase the expression of the adrenergic receptor, which promotes increased prostatic concentrations of DHT and reduces the rate of prostate cell death.[37-39] BPH can be induced in castrated dogs via supplementation with aromatizable androgens, and this effect can be blocked by concomitant administration of aromatase inhibitors that prevent conversion of testosterone to estrogen.[37,38] However, clinical studies using aromatase inhibitors (ie, atamestane, testolactone) as monotherapy for the treatment of BPH have failed to yield encouraging results.[40-42] The failure of aromatase inhibitors to improve BPH symptomatology may be related to a simultaneous rise in testosterone concentration leading to glandular epithelial hyperplasia of the prostate.[40-42]

### Adverse Effects of Hormonal Therapy

The most deleterious effects of agents altering the hypothalamic/adrenal/gonadal axis at different levels along the pathway are related to varying degrees of sexual dysfunction (Table 4-2). Interventions that markedly lower serum testosterone levels are associated with greater degrees of sexual dysfunction (eg, loss of libido) than are agents that block the effect of testosterone on target organs.[43]

## α-Adrenergic Antagonists

Symptomatic BPH results from two major components of prostate growth: static and dynamic. The dynamic component is associated with an increase in smooth muscle tone mediated by the autonomic nervous system. Prostatic smooth muscle cells contract under the influence of noradrenergic sympathetic nerves, and subsequently constrict the urethra and impair uroflow. In addition, there is recent evidence that adrenergic receptors mediate LUTS via their activation within the central nervous system (CNS) and bladder.[33,34] The prostate gland contains high levels of both $\alpha_1/\alpha_2$-adrenergic receptors.[44-47] However, the majority (about 98%) of the $\alpha_1$-adrenergic receptors are associated with the stromal elements of the prostate and subsequently have the largest influence on urethral tone. Thus, blockade of the $\alpha_1$-adrenergic receptor would be expected to relax prostatic smooth muscle, relieve bladder outlet obstruction (BOO), and enhance uroflow.

## Table 4-2: Adverse Effects of Hormonal Therapy

| Effect | 5ARI, Type 2 (finasteride), % |
|--------|-------------------------------|
| Impotence | 3-4 |
| Loss of libido | 4-5 |
| Ejaculatory dysfunction | 4-5 |
| Hot flashes | - |
| Gynecomastia | - |
| Diarrhea | - |

The promise for medical therapy using $\alpha$-adrenergic receptor blockers first emerged during the study of phenoxybenzamine (Dibenzyline®). Phenoxybenzamine is a nonselective $\alpha_1/\alpha_2$-receptor blocker found to be effective in relieving the symptoms of BPH.[48-51] However, side effects, such as dizziness, weakness, and palpitations, limited the use of this drug for BPH therapy. It was noticed that while both $\alpha_1/\alpha_2$-receptors were in the prostate, prostatic smooth muscle contraction was dominated by $\alpha_1$-receptors. Therefore, it was presumed that many of the adverse effects associated with this drug were induced by $\alpha_2$-receptor blockers. These findings led to the development of $\alpha_1$-selective blockers for the successful medical therapy of BPH.

These two different subtypes of $\alpha$-receptors ($\alpha_1$ and $\alpha_2$) are distributed ubiquitously throughout the human body. $\alpha_2$-Receptors are located presynaptically and cause

| 5ARI, Types 1 & 2 (dutasteride), % | GnRH Agonists, % | Anti-androgens, % |
|---|---|---|
| 1-6 | 95-100 | 10-20 |
| 4 | 95-100 | 10-20 |
| 1-2 | - | - |
| - | 95-100 | - |
| 1-2 | 0-5 | 50-100 |
| - | - | 50 |

5ARI=5α-reductase inhibitor; GnRH=gonadotropin-releasing hormone

down-regulation of norepinephrine release via a negative feedback mechanism. $\alpha_1$-Receptors are located postsynaptically and are targeted for the treatment of BPH.[45] Based on the molecular characterization, differential binding affinities, and cloning of unique DNA sequences, a number of subtypes of the $\alpha_1$-adrenergic receptors have been identified.[52,53] These subtypes have been classified into three groups: $\alpha_{1A}$, $\alpha_{1B}$, and $\alpha_{1D}$.[54]

Although both $\alpha_{1A}$ and $\alpha_{1B}$ are present in the prostate, $\alpha_{1A}$ is the predominant adrenergic receptor expressed by smooth muscle cells in this location (Table 4-3).[45] Therefore, blockade of the $\alpha_{1A}$-adrenergic receptors reduces prostatic tone and improves the dynamic aspects of voiding.[55] The $\alpha_{1D}$-subtype of adrenergic receptors is primarily located in the bladder body and dome. Detrusor instability appears to occur via stimulation of these receptors, and blockade of

## Table 4-3: Location of Different Subtypes of α-Adrenergic Receptors

| Location | $\alpha_{1A}$ | $\alpha_{1B}$ | $\alpha_{1D}$ |
|---|---|---|---|
| Bladder dome | + | + | +++ |
| Bladder trigone | +++ | + | + |
| Prostate gland | +++ | + | + |
| Prostatic urethra | +++ | + | + |
| Penile urethra | +++ | + | + |
| Vasculature | + | +++ | + |
| Spinal cord | + | + | +++ |

these receptors has been shown in animal models to reduce irritative voiding symptoms.[56] $\alpha_{1D}$-Receptors are also located in the spinal cord where they are presumed to play a role in the sympathetic modulation of parasympathetic activity.[57] The $\alpha_{1B}$-subtype of receptors are located in the smooth muscle of arteries and veins, including the microvasculature contained within the prostate gland.[54] Blockade of these receptors in the cardiovascular system causes symptoms of dizziness and hypotension due to decreased total peripheral resistance via veno- and arterial dilatation. This is a potentially serious side effect, as many patients who present with BPH also have co-existing comorbidities, such as coronary artery disease. Taken together, it appears that combined $\alpha_{1A}$- and $\alpha_{1D}$-receptor antagonist action is one of the best options for the management of BPH.

Based on this knowledge, pharmaceutical companies have developed multiple different α-adrenergic antagonists and, with more understanding and development, have been able to enhance their selectivity (Table 4-4).

## Table 4-4: Types and Characteristics of Different $\alpha$-Adrenergic Receptor Antagonists

| Name | Rank Order of Receptor Selectivity* |
|------|-------------------------------------|
| Prazosin (Minipress®, Minipress® XL) | $\alpha_{1A}=\alpha_{1B}=\alpha_{1D}$ |
| Doxazosin (Cardura®, Cardura® XL) | $\alpha_{1A}=\alpha_{1B}=\alpha_{1D}$ |
| Terazosin (Hytrin®) | $\alpha_{1B}=\alpha_{1D}>\alpha_{1A}$ |
| Alfuzosin (Uroxatral®) | $\alpha_{1A}=\alpha_{1B}=\alpha_{1D}$ |
| Tamsulosin (Flomax®) | $\alpha_{1A}=\alpha_{1D}>\alpha_{1B}$ |

*Adapted from Lyseng-Williamson et al[58]. Used with permission.

Recent terminology categorizes $\alpha$-blockers according to their action on specific subtypes of $\alpha$-adrenergic receptors. The original $\alpha$-blockers, such as phenoxybenzamine and prazosin, were discontinued because they antagonized both prostatic and vascular $\alpha_1$- and $\alpha_2$-adrenergic receptors, resulting in syncope, orthostatic hypotension, reflex tachycardia, cardiac arrhythmias, and retrograde ejaculation. The above drugs have been replaced in BPH treatment by the newer $\alpha$-blockers terazosin (Hytrin®), doxazosin (Cardura®, Cardura® XL), tamsulosin (Flomax®), and alfuzosin (Uroxatral®).

The $\alpha$-blockers used to treat BPH are further divided according to their ability to target the $\alpha_{1A}$-adrenergic receptor subtype of $\alpha_1$-adrenergic receptors. The nonuroselective $\alpha$-blockers, terazosin and doxazosin, target the $\alpha_1$-adrenergic

## Table 4-5: Adverse Effects of α-Adrenergic Receptor Antagonists[62-67]

| Effect | Phenoxy-benzamine, % | Prazosin, % |
|---|---|---|
| Hypotension | 15-20 | 10-15 |
| Dizziness | 10-14 | 15-17 |
| Headache | 4-15 | 13-15 |
| Erectile dysfunction (ED) | 5-8 | NR |
| Ejaculatory dysfunction | 2-10 | 5-20 |
| Fatigue | 10-15 | 10 |
| Syncope | NR | NR |
| Nasal congestion | 8 | NR |

NR=not recorded; phenoxybenzamine (Dibenzyline®)

receptors in the prostate gland. The uroselective α-blockers, tamsulosin and alfuzosin, achieve higher affinity and concentration in the prostate. Tamsulosin targets the $\alpha_{1A}$-adrenergic receptor, which is the predominant $\alpha_1$-adrenergic receptor subtype in the prostate (70%). Alfuzosin does not specifically target the $\alpha_1$-adrenergic receptor subtype, instead achieving its uroselectivity by its ability to attain higher tissues concentration.

### Terazosin, Doxazosin, Alfuzosin, and Tamsulosin

Terazosin (Table 4-5) is a relatively long-acting, non-uroselective α-blocker that allows for once-daily dosing.

| Tera-zosin, % | Doxa-zosin, % | Tamsulo-sin, % | Alfu-zosin, % |
|---|---|---|---|
| 2-8 | 1-2 | <1 | <1 |
| 7-14 | 10-15 | 15 | 6-9 |
| 4-10 | 9-10 | 19 | 8-14 |
| 2-7 | 2-8 | 2-10 | 1-5 |
| 0-1 | 0-1 | 8.4-18.1 | 0-1 |
| 4-8 | 1-2 | 8 | 1-7 |
| <1 | <1 | <1 | <1 |
| 2 | NR | 13 | 5-6 |

The Hytrin Community Assessment Trial (HCAT) is representative of the results obtained from many clinical trials of patients treated with terazosin.[59] The HCAT study enrolled 2,084 men ≥55 years with moderate-to-severe urinary symptoms and randomized them to receive treatment with terazosin (2 to 10 mg dose) or placebo. Terazosin was significantly superior to placebo in all measurements of efficacy in the trial; the AUA-IPSS score improved from a baseline mean of 20.1 points by 37.8% in the terazosin group, compared with 18.4% in the placebo group. The mean change from baseline in $Q_{max}$ was 2.2 for terazosin compared with 0.8 for placebo. Treatment failure occurred in about 11% of the terazosin study group, compared with about 25% in the placebo group. Withdrawal from the study due to adverse effects of treatment occurred in 20% of the terazosin study group. However, terazosin given once daily in community-based settings is an effective medical therapy for reducing LUTS and impairment of quality of life (QOL) due to urinary symptoms created by BPH.

Doxazosin (Table 4-5) is a long-acting, nonuroselective α-blocker that allows for once-daily dosing. Short-term clinical trials have demonstrated that doxazosin can increase $Q_{max}$ by about 1 to 4 mL/sec and decrease AUA symptom scores by up to 50% in men with symptomatic BPH. The clinical response to $\alpha_1$-receptor antagonists in terms of decreased symptomatology and increased uroflow rates is dose dependent; however, the side-effect profile is also dose dependent. Therefore, doxazosin therapy for BPH is typically initiated at a dose of 1 mg administered once daily. This low-starting dose is intended to minimize the frequency of side effects, such as postural hypotension and syncope. Depending on the patient's response to therapy and urodynamics, the dosage may be increased to 8 mg/day. Overall, doxazosin is an effective therapy for symptomatic BPH.[60-62] Like terazosin, it has been proven to relieve symptoms and improve uroflow rates.

Alfuzosin (Table 4-5) is a uroselective α-blocker indicated for the management of moderate-to-severe urinary symptoms due to BPH. Use of an extended-release (ER) formulation (10 mg once daily) for the treatment of the signs and symptoms of BPH was approved by the US Food and Drug Administration (FDA) in 2003 based on clinical trials showing improvement in irritative and obstructive urinary symptoms, as well as in $Q_{max}$, with alfuzosin ER compared with placebo.[63,64]

In a meta-analysis of three clinical trials, the vasodilatory adverse-event profile seen with alfuzosin ER 10 mg was similar to that with placebo, and, as in other studies of alfuzosin ER, the incidence of ejaculatory dysfunction or erectile dysfunction (ED) was low (<1%).[63,64] The three studies (which had similar study design, inclusion, and exclusion criteria) enrolled a total of 984 patients with BPH, who were randomized to receive either alfuzosin (n=473) or placebo (n=482) for 84 days. The number of study withdrawals was similar in both groups (placebo 42 [8.7%] vs alfuzosin 45 [9.5%]). No significant changes in blood pressure were observed with alfuzosin ER compared with placebo, hypotension, and syncope were uncommon, and no first-dose vasodilatory effect was seen, indicating that there is no need to titrate doses when initiating treatment with alfuzosin ER.[63,64] Data from the meta-analysis of three clinical trials also suggest that alfuzosin ER 10 mg helped to slow or prevent progression to more serious medical conditions; no patients given alfuzosin ER experienced AUR, compared with two patients who received placebo (0.4%).[63,64]

Data concerning the long-term efficacy and safety of the newer alfuzosin ER formulation are also beginning to emerge.[65] In a long-term (ie, 9 months), open-label extension of a 3-month double-blind, placebo-controlled trial in which all participants (N=311) received alfuzosin ER 10 mg; mean IPSS improved significantly, from 17.1 at baseline to 9.3 at end of study ($P$ <0.0001); and mean $Q_{max}$ rate increased from 9.1 to 11.3 mL/sec ($P$ <0.0001). In this study, 29 (9.3%) patients were discontinued from this phase of the study. The most frequent reason cited for discontinuation was adverse events (12/311 or 3.9%), while insufficient efficacy was cited in seven (7/311 or 2.3%) patients. Significant symptom relief was achieved rapidly with alfuzosin ER and was maintained at study end. Bother scores also improved significantly, from 3.3 at baseline to 2.1 at study end ($P$ <0.0001).

Until recently, sexual dysfunction in older men has been perceived as of secondary importance. However, there is now clear evidence that most men remain sexually active into their 70s,[36,37] and sexuality is an important component of QOL in men with symptomatic BPH.[38,39] Furthermore, there is a growing appreciation of the fact that LUTS is associated with an increased incidence of sexual dysfunction.[40-42]

A recent open-label study of 3,076 men treated with alfuzosin 10 mg for 1 year were assessed for the effect of treatment on sexual function.[68] Of the 3,076 men analyzed, 2,078 (67.6%) had completed 1 year of the study, 285 (9.3%) were ongoing, and 713 (23.2%) discontinued the study, primarily because of adverse events (238/3,076 or 7.7%) or insufficient efficacy (220/3,076 or 7.2%). In this population, reduced stiffness of erection, reduced volume of ejaculate, and pain/discomfort on ejaculation were reported at baseline by 65.3%, 63.2%, and 20.2% of participants, respectively. These data provide strong evidence that LUTS and/or BPH are directly associated with sexual dysfunction. At the study end point, the mean Danish Prostate Symptom Score (DAN-PSS) including the sexual function domain (DAN-PSSsex) scores for each of these symptoms improved significantly (all $P$ <0.001).[68] These improvements were apparent from the first assessment at 3 months and maintained throughout the study.[68] The study also found that alfuzosin was effective in the improvement of LUTS and QOL, and that it may even improve sexual function in those men with concomitant ED and/or ejaculatory dysfunction.

It should be noted that this apparent improvement in sexual dysfunction is not associated with other α-adrenergic blocking agents. For example, tamsulosin, the other uroselective α-blocker, is associated with an increased incidence of ejaculatory dysfunction ranging from 8.4% (0.4 mg) to 18.1% (0.8 mg) of patients.[66] The mechanism of these different effects on sexual dysfunction remains to be clarified.

With long-term use of alfuzosin, lasting improvements in sexuality and health-related QOL have been consistently observed.[64-68] For example, in their 3-year follow-up of patients, Lukacs and colleagues demonstrated improvements in patient sexuality using the UroLife BPH-QOL scale.[69] Specifically, with up to 3 years of alfuzosin treatment, improvements in sexual life subscores were seen among patients of all ages, with the greatest degree of sexual improvement occurring among those patients who reported severe symptoms at baseline, regardless of age.[69] Other studies[64-68] indicate that alfuzosin is not likely to interfere with sexual function by giving rise to unwanted sexual side effects, such as ejaculatory dysfunction or ED. Clinical trials have shown that ejaculatory dysfunction and ED with alfuzosin are infrequent (0.0% to 0.6%), and, in most cases, are judged by investigators not to be related to treatment.[64-68] These and other studies also indicate that long-term alfuzosin therapy tends to have a positive impact on patient BPH-related QOL and bother associated with symptoms.[64-69]

Community-based investigations of the natural history of BPH and LUTS due to BPH indicate that, left untreated, the disease progresses over time with variable frequency.[4] In a large, 5-year prospective investigation, it was found that men with moderate LUTS due to BPH who underwent watchful waiting had poorer outcomes than those who received treatment (ie, transurethral resection of the prostate [TURP]), with significantly higher incidences observed for AUR, high residual urine volume, and severe LUTS.[45] However, risk of renal impairment appears remote.[46] Moreover, receipt of treatment only after the appearance of complications or worsening symptoms was associated with poorer response to treatment, suggesting the possible presence of irreversible damage.[45]

In line with these data, some evidence suggests that pharmacotherapy with alfuzosin may also alter the natural history of BPH-related urinary symptoms and reduce certain complications (ie, AUR).[64-69] In a 2-year, open-label extension of a placebo-controlled study (N=72),

Jardin et al[70,71] found that patients who received alfuzosin therapy did not show any signs of BPH disease-related deterioration (eg, bladder infection, AUR). A number of other long-term, open-label investigations have demonstrated a lower incidence of AUR with alfuzosin treatment, compared with the historical rates seen with watchful waiting.[64-69] For instance, in the 3-year prospective, open-label study of alfuzosin IR (2.5 mg three times daily) by Lukacs et al,[69] there was an extremely low incidence (0.3%) of AUR episodes overall, which is dramatically lower than the 2.9% overall rate seen in another investigation among patients with moderate BPH treated only with watchful waiting. Admittedly, such cross-study comparison involves different patient cohorts, but the sharply lower incidence of AUR seen with alfuzosin between two similar groups of patients suggests that this difference is not spurious.

With recent shifts in treatment practices, patients with LUTS due to BPH are likely to receive pharmacotherapy over long periods. Symptom relief with $\alpha_1$-blockers such as alfuzosin has been well established in short-term clinical trials. Alfuzosin administration in doses ranging from 7.5 to 10 mg/day is consistently associated with rapid symptom improvement. Findings from studies of long-term alfuzosin use demonstrate positive medical and personal outcomes in patients treated with this agent.

Examination of the efficacy and safety of long-term use of alfuzosin also shows that this compound's therapeutic effects on BPH-related symptoms are persistent, with no evidence of a waning response over a treatment period of 3 years. With longer term use, positive effects on health-related QOL and sexual functioning also tend to emerge and appear to be persistent. Other data suggest that long-term management of BPH-related symptoms with alfuzosin, particularly alfuzosin-related decreases in postvoid residual urine (PVR) volume, may help to decrease the incidence of spontaneous AUR and other BPH-related complications in this patient population. Moreover, acute treatment with alfuzosin may improve rates of spontaneous micturition in patients experiencing an initial episode of AUR. Continued study of the long-term use of alfuzosin is needed to obtain additional information concerning BPH symptom management and patient health outcomes.

Tamsulosin (Table 4-5) is a newer, uroselective α-blocker with specificity for the $\alpha_{1A}$-adrenergic receptor in relation to the $\alpha_{1B}$-adrenergic receptor.[72] Therefore, this drug should selectively target the smooth muscle cells contained within the prostate gland and exert minimal effects on the other α-adrenergic receptor subtypes that regulate blood-pressure control and vasodilation. Clinical trials suggest that tamsulosin provides relatively rapid action onset, based upon symptom improvement and $Q_{max}$. The initial short-term clinical trials suggested that tamsulosin increases $Q_{max}$ approximately 1.5 mL/sec and decreased AUA-IPSS by >35%.[73,74] Long-term studies (up to 60 weeks) examining the effects of tamsulosin demonstrate that its beneficial effects are sustained over time, as measured by $Q_{max}$ and AUA symptom scores. Tamsulosin was tolerated during the study period, with side effects occurring in about 21% of patients. The most common side effects reported with tamsulosin use are dizziness (about 14.9%) and retrograde ejaculation (about 8.4%). Clinical studies have also demonstrated that tamsulosin can be co-administered with antihypertensive medications such as atenolol (Tenormin®), enalapril (Vasotec®), and nifedipine (Procardia®, Procardia® XL) without any increased risk of hypotensive or syncopal episodes.[73,74] Taken together, tamsulosin is a safe and efficacious drug for the treatment of BPH without major vascular side effects.[73,74]

### Adverse Effects Associated with α-Adrenergic Antagonists

Depending on dosage and selectivity, all α-adrenergic antagonists can be associated with adverse reactions (Table 4-5).[62-67] Dizziness is the most common side effect of $\alpha$-adrenergic antagonists, possibly caused by effects upon the CNS or other unconventional drug mechanisms potentially unrelated to effects on the blood vessels themselves. The fact that some dizziness is seen with tamsulosin (a selective $\alpha_{1A}$-adrenergic antagonist) suggests a central effect may mediate this symptom. Hypotension decreases with longer acting drugs and occurs least with $\alpha_{1A}$-adrenergic selective agents. Dizziness and hypotension are more common in those over 65 years. Ejaculatory dysfunction may occur, but when explained to the patient, does not generally cause a problem. The adverse side effects of $\alpha$-adrenergic antagonists are mediated through drug interactions with the vas deferens itself.

## Combination Therapy

As mentioned above, both hormonal therapy and $\alpha$-adrenergic therapy are effective treatments for symptomatic BPH. The hormonal therapy is generally believed to target the static component, while the $\alpha$-adrenergic therapy is directed toward the dynamic component of BPH. Based on this assumption, it was believed combination therapy could target both the major components of BPH simultaneously.

The first randomized, double-blind, placebo-controlled study investigating combination therapy using $\alpha$-adrenergic antagonists and 5ARIs was the four-arm Veterans Administration Cooperative (VA COOP) study comparing placebo, finasteride alone, terazosin alone, and combination therapy with finasteride and terazosin.[75] After 1 year of treatment, the investigators concluded that short-term combination therapy was no more effective than a single agent in the treatment of BPH. Terazosin alone produced superior results in terms of improvement of AUA symptom scores and $Q_{max}$. Treatment with finasteride showed the most significant decrease in prostate size, but reports of bothersome symptoms did not correspond. A subsequent clinical trial, known as the Prospective European Doxazosin and Combined Therapy (PREDICT) trial, also examined whether combination therapy with $\alpha$-adrenergic inhibitors and 5ARIs could be used for the symptomatic treatment of BPH.[61] The conclusions of this study confirmed that the $\alpha$-adrenergic inhibitor, doxazosin, was a superior treatment for symptomatic BPH compared with finasteride alone or placebo. The addition of finasteride to doxazosin did not provide any increased benefit compared with doxazosin alone.

The applicability of the study's conclusion to the general population of men with symptomatic BPH was subsequently challenged due to the relatively small percentage of participants with larger prostates. It also failed to address whether combination therapy affected BPH progression or whether longer duration of therapy affected the outcome.

The Medical Treatment of Prostatic Symptoms (MTOPS) study was a four-arm clinical trial (placebo, doxazosin, finasteride, combination) that revisited the utility of combination therapy.[76,77] The study leaders questioned whether combination therapy could prevent clinical disease progression by treatment with finasteride, doxazosin, or both.[77] The investigators followed a total of 3,047 men for 4.5 years. The study participants all had relatively large prostate volumes (average of 36.5 mL) at the beginning of the study. The clinical outcomes that were measured included the incidence of AUR, renal insufficiency, recurrent urinary tract infections (UTIs), and changes in AUA-IPSS.

The MTOPS study clearly demonstrated that, compared with monotherapy, there was a significant risk reduction in the progression of BPH with combination therapy. This risk reduction included a sustained measurable decrease in AUA-IPSS, a decreased risk of developing AUR, and a decreased incidence of surgical treatment for BPH (Table 4-6).

One way to assess BPH progression is by documenting an increase in AUA-IPSS. The MTOPS study demonstrated that an increase in AUA-IPSS of >4 points above baseline values was the most common individual adverse event in all groups at the end of the study. In fact, there was a 3.6/100 person-years risk of having this 4-point

**Table 4-6:** **Risk of BPH Progression as Measured by AUA-IPSS, Rates of AUR, and Requirement for Surgical Intervention: Doxazosin vs Finasteride vs Combination Therapy[77]**

| Therapy | Risk Reduction in Increasing AUA-IPSS |
|---|---|
| Doxazosin | 45% |
| Finasteride | 30% |
| Combination therapy (finasteride + doxazosin) | 66% |

AUA-IPSS=American Urological Association-International Prostate Symptom Scores; AUR=acute urinary retention; BPH=benign prostatic hypertension

increase in the placebo arm of the study. In comparison, the risk of having a 4-point increase in AUA-IPSS was reduced to 1.9 person-years (45% reduction in risk) in the doxazosin group. Similarly, patients in the finasteride group had a 30% reduction in risk. Patients enrolled in the combination therapy arm of the study experienced a 66% reduction in the risk of higher AUA-IPSS. In fact, this risk reduction was larger than any of the medical therapies used alone.

The MTOPS study also analyzed the contribution of monotherapy and combination therapy toward the incidence of AUR.[77] Doxazosin did not significantly reduce the rate of AUR compared with the placebo group (0.4/100 person-years). However, both the finasteride monotherapy (0.4/100 person-years) and combination therapy (0.1/100 person-years) groups significantly lowered the rate of development of urinary retention compared with the

| Risk Reduction in Urinary Retention | Risk Reduction for Requiring Surgical Treatment |
|---|---|
| 35% | 3% |
| 68% | 64% |
| 81% | 67% |

placebo group (0.6/100 person-years). The table depicted above demonstrates an insignificant decrease of 35% in the doxazosin group, and a significant decrease of 68% and 81% in the finasteride monotherapy and combination therapy groups, respectively.

The MTOPS study also demonstrated a significant reduction in the rate of invasive surgical treatment over a 5-year period when either finasteride monotherapy or combination therapy with finasteride and doxazosin is used.[77] Men enrolled in the placebo group had a 1.3/100 person-years risk of having invasive surgery for BPH (such as transurethral prostatectomy or transurethral microwave thermotherapy [TUMT]). The risk of requiring these invasive treatments for progression of BPH was reduced by 64% and 67% in the finasteride and combination therapy groups, respectively. Doxazosin did not significantly reduce the incidence of invasive treatments.

## Table 4-7: Adverse Effects of Combination Therapy for BPH *

| Effect | Placebo |
| --- | --- |
| Hypotension | 2.29 |
| Dizziness | 2.29 |
| Asthenia | 2.06 |
| ED | 3.32 |
| Decreased libido | 1.40 |
| Abnormal ejaculation | 0.83 |
| Allergic reaction | 0.46 |

BPH=benign prostatic hyperplasia; ED=erectile dysfunction

*Adverse reactions reported in 100 person-years of follow-up.

Adapted from McConnell et al[77]

As mentioned above, the MTOPS trial demonstrated a decrease in the progression of BPH associated with combination therapy with finasteride and doxazosin. Since the initiation of MTOPS, studies have shown that patients with larger prostates and higher prostate-specific antigen (PSA) levels are at increased risk for BPH progression, and are therefore arguably more likely to benefit from combination therapy. The Combination of Avodart and Tamsulosin (CombAT) trial is an ongoing 4-year, multicenter, randomized, double-blind study designed to investigate the benefits of combination therapy with the $5\alpha$-reductase inhibitor, dutasteride, and the $\alpha$-blocker, tamsulosin, compared with each monotherapy in improving symptoms and long-term outcomes in men with moderate-to-severe LUTS due to BPH.[78] The study involves 4,800 men, and of the men studied, 1,492 were treated with a combination of dutasteride

| Doxazosin | Finasteride | Combination |
|-----------|-------------|-------------|
| 4.03 | 2.56 | 4.33 |
| 4.41 | 2.33 | 5.35 |
| 4.08 | 1.56 | 4.20 |
| 3.56 | 4.53 | 5.11 |
| 1.56 | 2.36 | 2.51 |
| 1.10 | 1.78 | 3.05 |
| 0.85 | 0.58 | 0.73 |

and tamsulosin, 1,502 were prescribed dutasteride alone, and 1,519 were prescribed tamsulosin alone. Eligible patients are ≥50 years with an estimated prostate volume ≥30 cm³ and PSA level ≥1.5 ng/mL. In pivotal 2-year phase 3 trials, oral dutasteride 0.5 mg once daily improved urinary symptoms, decreased total prostate volume (TPV), and reduced the risk of AUR and BPH-related surgery in men with moderate-to-severe symptoms of BPH and prostate enlargement.[79] The efficacy and tolerability of dutasteride was maintained for up to 4 years in open-label extension studies. Results of the preplanned, 2-year interim analysis of the CombAT trial showed that the combination of dutasteride and tamsulosin was superior to either drug as monotherapy in improving BPH-related symptoms, $Q_{max}$, and BPH-related health status. In another analysis of CombAT trial data, Roehrborn et al[80] concluded that men with moderate-to-severe LUTS and prostate enlargement (ie, $\geq$30 mL) combination therapy provides a significantly greater degree of benefit than tamsulosin or dutasteride monotherapy.

## Adverse Effects of Combination Therapy for Benign Prostatic Hyperplasia

As mentioned in prior sections, patients assigned to the doxazosin group had an increased rate of dizziness and postural hypotension compared with patients enrolled in the placebo group. Similarly, ED, decreased libido, and abnormal ejaculation had a higher frequency rate compared with placebo. The adverse events experienced by patients taking combination therapy were similar to those for each drug alone. However, the rates of abnormal ejaculation, peripheral edema, and dyspnea were increased in this group (Table 4-7).[77]

## Other Combination Therapy

### LUTS and Overactive Bladder

It is known that chronic BOO alters the cellular content of the bladder and affects detrusor behavior. Many times, men with BOO due to BPH will develop LUTS that includes detrusor hyperactivity. Traditionally, patients with symptoms related to overactive bladder (OAB) are treated with antimuscarinic agents to inhibit bladder contractility. However, when questioned, men with detrusor hyperactivity and LUTS did not respond to monotherapy with either antimuscarinic agents or $\alpha$-receptor antagonists. Recent evidence suggests that combination therapy with a antimuscarinic agent and an $\alpha$-receptor antagonist may provide some benefit.[81] For example, a randomized, double-blind, placebo-controlled trial conducted at 95 urology clinics in the United States involving men $\geq$40 years who reported moderate-to-severe LUTS and a bladder diary documenting micturition frequency ($\geq$8 micturitions per 24 hours) and urgency ($\geq$3 episodes per 24 hours), with or without urgency urinary incontinence, were randomly assigned to receive placebo (n=222), an antimuscarinic agent (tolterodine ER [n=217], Detrol LA®), an α-receptor antagonist (tamsulosin [n=215]), or both (n=225) for 12 weeks. The results suggested that patients receiving both tolterodine ER and tamsulosin experienced significant reductions in urinary urgency symptoms and incontinence compared with placebo ($P=0.005$). These improvements were experienced in addition to significant improvements in LUTS. There was a low rate of AUR with combination therapy (0.4%). This study provides evidence that combination therapy may provide benefits for men with moderate-to-severe LUTS, including OAB due to BPH.

## LUTS and Erectile Dysfunction

There is emerging evidence of a strong relationship between symptomatic BPH and ED.[82] While the exact mechanism linking these two conditions has not been elucidated, it is hypothesized they share a common pathophysiology. A number of theories exist to suggest this association, including one theory based upon decreased nitric oxide (NO) production within the penis, bladder, and prostate gland.[82] NO is a molecule released from neuronal and endothelial structures known to be involved in the relaxation of the corpus cavernosum smooth muscle and vasculature. Conditions associated with reduced function of nerves and endothelium include aging, hypertension, smoking, and diabetes (all conditions associated with ED). Thus, decreased production of NO within the prostate and erectile tissues may manifest as ED and LUTS comorbidities.

Recent studies suggest that the phosphodiesterase inhibitor-5 (PDE-5) may be beneficial for more than just the treatment of ED. Recently, a randomized, controlled phase II trial of the PDE-5 tadalafil (Cialis®) vs placebo for the treatment of symptomatic BPH revealed that tadalafil had statistically significant and clinically meaningful efficacy in both the treatment of ED and the treatment of LUTS due to BPH.[83,84] In another recent study, it was reported that sildenafil (Viagra®) improves AUA

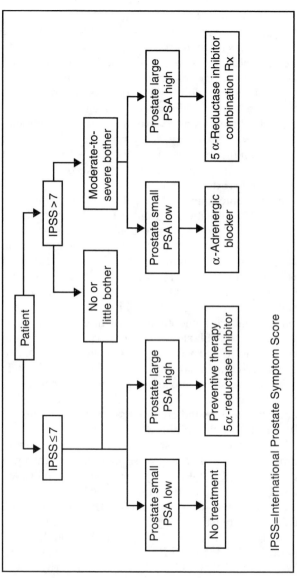

IPSS=International Prostate Symptom Score

**Figure 4-3:** Algorithm for the medical management of BPH.

symptom scores.[85] In addition, it has also been reported that treatment with α-adrenergic antagonists can relieve chronic ED. It should be noted that PDE-5 may potentiate hypotension in patients who are on α-adrenergic antagonists for the treatment of LUTS due to BPH. While the FDA has recently approved the concomitant use of these drugs, caution should be exercised and the patient should understand this risk.

## Algorithm for the Medical Management of BPH

BPH is a common complaint that increases with aging. As the prostate enlarges, it can cause clinical symptoms because it obstructs the urinary outlet by its larger physical size (static component) and increased smooth muscle tone (dynamic component). Treatment intervention for clinical BPH has mostly been directed toward the alleviation of bothersome LUTS. However, more recent attention has been focused on the prevention of BPH related to disease progression.

Watchful waiting is an appropriate option for patients who present with mild LUTS (AUA-IPSS ≤7). As the name implies, this strategy does not involve any therapy and requires annual reassessment of a patient's symptoms. The patient should be taught behavioral techniques to reduce symptoms, such as limiting nighttime fluid intake.

Individual patient probabilities of BPH progression are difficult to predict. However, it should be noted that symptoms related to BPH progress in many patients and the ability to predict progression depends on the initial presentation of symptoms. For example, in the Olmsted County Study of Urinary Symptoms and Health Status Among Men, over a 4-year period, about 67% of men who presented with mild urinary symptoms experienced worsened symptoms (50% progressed to moderate symptoms, 7% to severe symptoms, and 10% chose surgery). Forty-one percent of men who presented initially with moderate symptoms progressed to severe symptoms and 24% underwent surgery. Thirty-nine percent of patients with severe symptoms at the initial time of observation chose surgery over a 4-year period. If a patient's symptoms progress to moderate or severe levels, it is appropriate to reassess the situation and offer treatment modalities.

The decision to institute medical therapy for BPH begins with an appropriate assessment and examination of the patient. In the United States, the finding of a small, smooth prostate in an individual with moderate or severe LUTS invokes the use of an α-adrenergic receptor antagonist (Figure 4-3). Combination therapy with an α-adrenergic receptor antagonist and a 5ARI should be used for patients who present with bothersome LUTS and a large prostate (>50 g). This combination therapy is directed at relieving acute LUTS as well as preventing BPH progression (Table 4-7). In addition, it is now suggested that patients with mild or no symptoms, but who have a large prostate, should be started on monotherapy with a 5ARI to prevent BPH progression. The role of therapy with an α-adrenergic receptor antagonist combined with either an antimuscarinic agent or a PDE-5 has not been reviewed by the AUA. However, these therapies may be considered for patients with moderate-to-severe LUTS associated with either ED or symptoms of urinary urgency.

## References

1. Lee C, Kozlowski JM, Grayhack JT: Etiology of benign prostatic hyperplasia. *Urol Clin North Am* 1995;22:237-246.

2. Lee C, Kozlowski, JM, Grayhack JT: Intrinsic and extrinsic factors controlling benign prostatic growth. *Prostate* 1997;31: 131-138.

3. Gosling JA, Dixon JS: Structure of trabeculated detrusor smooth muscle in cases of prostatic hypertrophy. *Urol Int* 1980;35: 351-355.

4. Di Silverio F, Genitle V, Pastore AL, et al: Benign prostatic hyperplasia: what about a campaign for prevention? *Urol Int* 2004; 72:179-188.

5.  O'Leary MP: Lower urinary tract symptoms/benign prostatic hyperplasia: maintaining symptom control and reducing complications. *Urology* 2003;62(3 suppl 1):15-23.

6.  Baine WB, Yu W, Summe JP, et al: Epidemiologic trends in the evaluation and treatment of lower urinary tract symptoms in elderly male Medicare patients from 1991 to 1995. *J Urol* 1998;160(3 pt 1): 816-820.

7.  Xia Z, Roberts RO, Schottenfeld D, et al: Trends in prostatectomy for benign prostatic hyperplasia among black and white men in the United States: 1980 to 1994. *Urology* 1999;53:1154-1159.

8.  Wasson JH, Bubolz TA, Lu-Yao GL, et al: Transurethral resection of the prostate among medicare beneficiaries: 1984 to 1997. For the Patient Outcomes Research Team for Prostatic Diseases. *J Urol* 2000;164:1212-1215.

9.  Partin, AW: *Etiology of Benign Prostatic Hyperplasia*. Philadelphia, PA, WB Saunders Co, 2000, pp 95-100.

10.  Isaacs JT, Coffey DS: Changes in dihydrotestosterone metabolism associated with the development of canine benign prostatic hyperplasia. *Endocrinology* 1981;108:445-453.

11.  Brooks JR, Berman D, Glitzer MS, et al: Effect of a new 5 alpha-reductase inhibitor on size, histologic characteristics, and androgen concentrations of the canine prostate. *Prostate* 1982;3: 35-44.

12.  McConnell JD, Akakura K, Bartsch G, et al: Hormonal treatment of benign prostatic hyperplasia. Paris, France, Scientific Communication International 1993, p 417.

13.  Geller J: Effect of finasteride, a 5 alpha-reductase inhibitor on prostate tissue androgens and prostate-specific antigen. *J Clin Endocrinol Metab* 1990;71:1552-1555.

14.  Vermeulen A, Giagulli VA, De Schepper P, et al: Hormonal effects of a 5 alpha-reductase inhibitor (finasteride) on hormonal levels in normal men and in patients with benign prostatic hyperplasia. *Eur Urol* 1991;20(suppl 1):82-86.

15.  McConnell JD, Wilson JD, George FW et al: Finasteride, an inhibitor of 5 alpha-reductase, suppresses prostatic dihydrotestosterone in men with benign prostatic hyperplasia. *J Clin Endocrinol Metab* 1992;74:505-508.

16.   Gormley GJ, Stoner E, Bruskewitz RC, et al: The effect of finasteride in men with benign prostatic hyperplasia. The Finasteride Study Group. *N Engl J Med* 1992;327:1185-1191.

17.   McConnell JD, Bruskewitz R, Walsh P, et al: The effect on finasteride on the risk of acute urinary retention and the need for surgical treatment among men with benign prostatic hyperplasia. Finasteride Long-Term Efficacy and Safety Study Group. *N Engl J Med* 1998;338:557-563.

18.   Boyle P, Gould AL, Roehrborn CG: Prostate volume predicts outcome of treatment of benign prostatic hyperplasia with finasteride: meta-analysis of randomized clinical trials. *Urology* 1996;48: 398-405.

19.   Lieber MM, Jacobsen SJ, Roberts RO, et al: Prostate volume and prostate-specific antigen in the absence of prostate cancer: a review of the relationship and prediction of long-term outcomes. *Prostate* 2001;49:208-212.

20.   Oesterling JE, Jacobsen SJ, Chute CG, et al: Serum prostate-specific antigen in a community-based population of healthy men. Establishment of age-specific reference ranges. *JAMA* 1993;270: 860-864.

21.   Guess HA, Heyse JF, Gormley GJ: The effect of finasteride on prostate-specific antigen in men with benign prostatic hyperplasia. *Prostate* 1993;22:31-37.

22.   Guess HA, Heyse JF, Gormley GJ, et al: Effect of finasteride on serum PSA concentration in men with benign prostatic hyperplasia. Results from the North American phase III clinical trial. *Urol Clin North Am* 1993;20:627-636.

23.   Lange PH: Is the prostate pill finally here? *N Engl J Med* 1992; 327:1234-1236.

24.   Stoner E: Three-year safety and efficacy data on the use of finasteride in the treatment of benign prostatic hyperplasia. *Urology* 1994;43:284-292; discussion 292-294.

25.   Oesterling JE, Roy J, Agha A, et al: Biologic variability of prostate-specific antigen and its usefulness as a marker for prostate cancer: effects of finasteride. The Finasteride PSA Study Group. *Urology* 1997;50:13-18.

26.   Thompson IM, Goodman PJ, Tangen CM, et al: The influence of finasteride on the development of prostate cancer. *N Engl J Med* 2003;349:215-224.

27.  Thompson IM, Tangen C, Goodman P: The Prostate Cancer Prevention Trial: design, status, and promise. *World J Urol* 2003;21: 28-30.

28.  Gisleskog PO, Hermann D, Hammarlund-Udenaes M, et al: A model for the turnover of dihydrotestosterone in the presence of the irreversible 5 alpha-reductase inhibitors GI198745 and finasteride. *Clin Pharmacol Ther* 1998;64:636-647.

29.  Shirakawa T, Okada H, Acharya B, et al: Messenger RNA levels and enzyme activities of 5 alpha-reductase types 1 and 2 in human benign prostatic hyperplasia (BPH) tissue. *Prostate* 2004;58: 33-40.

30.  Thigpen AE, Davis DL, Milatovich A, et al: Molecular genetics of steroid 5 alpha-reductase 2 deficiency. *J Clin Invest* 1992;90: 799-809.

31.  Evans HC, Goa KL: Dutasteride. *Drugs Aging* 2003;20:905-916; discussion 917-918.

32.  Roehrborn CG, Boyle P, Nickel JC, et al: Efficacy and safety of a dual inhibitor of 5-alpha-reductase types 1 and 2 (dutasteride) in men with benign prostatic hyperplasia. *Urology* 2002;60: 434-441.

33.  Roehrborn CG, Marks LS, Fenter T, et al: Efficacy and safety of dutasteride in the four-year treatment of men with benign prostatic hyperplasia. *Urology* 2004;63:709-715.

34.  Roehrborn CG, Lukkarinen O, Mark S, et al: Long-term sustained improvement in symptoms of benign prostatic hyperplasia with the dual 5alpha-reductase inhibitor dutasteride: results of 4-year studies. *BJU Int* 2005;96:572-577.

35.  Eri LM, Tveter KJ: A prospective, placebo-controlled study of the luteinizing hormone-releasing hormone agonist leuprolide as treatment for patients with benign prostatic hyperplasia. *J Urol* 1993;150(2 pt 1):359-364.

36.  Coffey DS, Walsh PC: Clinical and experimental studies of benign prostatic hyperplasia. *Urol Clin North Am* 1990;17:461-475.

37.  Barrack ER, Berry SJ: DNA synthesis in the canine prostate: effects of androgen and estrogen treatment. *Prostate* 1987;10:45-56.

38.  Berry SJ, Strandberg JD, Saunders WJ, et al: Development of canine benign prostatic hyperplasia with age. *Prostate* 1986;9: 363-373.

**4**

39.   Moore RJ, Gazak JM, Wilson JD: Regulation of cytoplasmic dihydrotestosterone binding in dog prostate by 17 beta-estradiol. *J Clin Invest* 1979;63:351-357.

40.   el Etreby MF: Atamestane: an aromatase inhibitor for the treatment of benign prostatic hyperplasia. A short review. *J Steroid Biochem Mol Biol* 1993;44:565-572.

41.   Habenicht UF, Tunn UW, Senge T, et al: Management of benign prostatic hyperplasia with particular emphasis on aromatase inhibitors. *J Steroid Biochem Mol Biol* 1993;44:557-563.

42.   Tunn UW, Goldschmidt AJ: [Aromatase inhibitors in the medical treatment of benign prostatic hypertrophy]. *J Urol (Paris)* 1993;99:307.

43.   Uroxatral® Package Insert. sanofi-aventis U.S. LLC, Bridgewater, NJ, 2007.

44.   Furuya S, Kumamoto Y, Yokoyama E, et al: Alpha-adrenergic activity and urethral pressure in prostatic zone in benign prostatic hypertrophy. *J Urol* 1982;128:836-839.

45.   Kobayashi S, Tang R, Shapiro E, et al: Characterization and localization of prostatic alpha 1 adrenoceptors using radioligand receptor binding on slide-mounted tissue section. *J Urol* 1993;150:2002-2006.

46.   Lepor H, Laddu A: Terazosin in the treatment of benign prostatic hyperplasia: the United States experience. *Br J Urol* 1992;70 (suppl 1):2-9.

47.   Yokoyama E, Furuya S, Kumamoto Y: [Quantitation of alpha-1 and beta adrenergic receptor densities in the human normal and hypertrophied prostate]. *Nippon Hinyokika Gakkai Zasshi* 1985;76:325-337.

48.   Abrams P, Hollister P, Lawrence J, et al: Bladder outflow obstruction treated with phenoxybenzamine. Preliminary note. *Br J Urol* 1982;54:530.

49.   Caine M, Perlberg S, Meretyk S: A placebo-controlled double-blind study of the effect of phenoxybenzamine in benign prostatic obstruction. *Br J Urol* 1978;50:551-554.

50.   Caine M, Perlberg S, Meretyk S: A placebo-controlled double-blind study of the effect of phenoxybenzamine in benign prostatic obstruction. 1978. *J Urol* 2002;167(2 pt 2):1101.

51. Caine M, Perlberg S, Shapiro A: Phenoxybenzamine for benign prostatic obstruction. Review of 200 cases. *Urology* 1981;17: 542-546.

52. Lepor H: Alpha blockade for the treatment of benign prostatic hyperplasia. *Urol Clin North Am* 1995;22:375-386.

53. Lepor H: Long-term efficacy and safety of terazosin in patients with benign prostatic hyperplasia. Terazosin Research Group. *Urology* 1995;45:406-413.

54. Price DT, Schwinn DA, Lomasney JW, et al: Identification, quantification, and localization of mRNA for three distinct alpha 1 adrenergic receptor subtypes in human prostate. *J Urol* 1993;150 (2 pt 1):546-551.

55. Beduschi MC, Beduschi R, Oesterling JE: Alpha-blockade therapy for benign prostatic hyperplasia: from a nonselective to a more selective alpha1A-adrenergic antagonist. *Urology* 1998;51:861-872.

56. Malloy BJ, Price DT, Price RR, et al: Alpha1-adrenergic receptor subtypes in human detrusor. *J Urol* 1998;160(3 pt 1): 937-943.

57. Smith MS, Schambra UB, Wilson KH, et al: Alpha1-adrenergic receptors in human spinal cord: specific localized expression of mRNA encoding alpha1-adrenergic receptor subtypes at four distinct levels. *Brain Res Mol Brain Res* 1999;63:254-261.

58. Lyseng-Williamson KA, Jarvis B, Wagstaff AJ: Tamsulosin: an update of its role in the management of lower urinary tract symptoms. *Drugs* 2002;62:135-167.

59. Roehrborn CG, Oesterling JE, Auerbach S, et al: The Hytrin Community Assessment Trial study: a one-year study of terazosin versus placebo in the treatment of men with symptomatic benign prostatic hyperplasia. HYCAT Investigator Group. *Urology* 1996;47: 159-168.

60. Kirby RS: Doxazosin in benign prostatic hyperplasia: effects on blood pressure and urinary flow in normotensive and hypertensive men. *Urology* 1995;46:182-186.

61. Kirby RS, Roehrborn C, Boyle P, et al: Efficacy and tolerability of doxazosin and finasteride, alone or in combination, in treatment of symptomatic benign prostatic hyperplasia: the Prospective European Doxazosin and Combination Therapy (PREDICT) trial. *Urology* 2003;61:119-126.

62. Roehrborn CG, Siegel RL: Safety and efficacy of doxazosin in benign prostatic hyperplasia: a pooled analysis of three double-blind, placebo-controlled studies. *Urology* 1996;48:406-415.

63. Roehrborn CG: Efficacy and safety of once-daily alfuzosin in the treatment of lower urinary tract symptoms and clinical benign prostatic hyperplasia: a randomized, placebo-controlled trial. *Urology* 2001;58:953-959.

64. Roehrborn CG, Van Kerrebroeck P, Nordling J: Safety and efficacy of alfuzosin 10 mg once-daily in the treatment of lower urinary tract symptoms and clinical benign prostatic hyperplasia: a pooled analysis of three double-blind, placebo-controlled studies. *BJU Int* 2003;92:257-261.

65. van Kerrebroeck P, Jardin A, Laval KU, et al: Efficacy and safety of a new prolonged release formulation of alfuzosin 10 mg once daily versus alfuzosin 2.5 mg thrice daily and placebo in patients with symptomatic benign prostatic hyperplasia. ALFORTI Study Group. *Eur Urol* 2000;37:306-313.

66. Dunn CJ, Matheson A, Faulds DM: Tamsulosin: a review of its pharmacology and therapeutic efficacy in the management of lower urinary tract symptoms. *Drugs Aging* 2002;19:135-161.

67. Wilt TJ, Howe W, MacDonald R: Terazosin for treating symptomatic benign prostatic obstruction: a systematic review of efficacy and adverse effects. *BJU Int* 2002;89:214-225.

68. van Moorselaar RJ, Hartung R, Emberton M, et al, and the ALF-ONE Study Group: Alfuzosin 10 mg once daily improves sexual function in men with lower urinary tract symptoms and concomitant sexual dysfunction. *BJU Int* 2005;95:603-608.

69. Lukacs B, Grange JC, Comet D, et al: History of 7,093 patients with lower urinary tract symptoms related to benign prostatic hyperplasia treated with alfuzosin in general practice up to 3 years. *Eur Urol* 2000;37:183-190.

70. Jardin A, Bensadoun H, Delauche-Cavallier MC, et al: Long-term treatment of benign prostatic hyperplasia with alfuzosin: a 12-18 month assessment. BPHALF Group. *Br J Urol* 1993;72 (5 pt 1):615-620.

71. Jardin A, Bensadoun H, Delauche-Cavallier MC, et al: Long-term treatment of benign prostatic hyperplasia with alfuzosin: a 24-30 month survey. BPHALF Group. *Br J Urol* 1994;74:579-584.

72. Abrams P, Schulman CC, Vaage S: Tamsulosin, a selective alpha 1c-adrenoceptor antagonist: a randomized, controlled trial in patients with benign prostatic 'obstruction' (symptomatic BPH). The European Tamsulosin Study Group. *Br J Urol* 1995;76: 325-336.

73. Michel MC, Mehlburger L, Bressel HU, et al: Comparison of tamsulosin efficacy in subgroups of patients with lower urinary tract symptoms. *Prostate Cancer Prostatic Dis* 1998;1:332-335.

74. Michel MC, Mehlburger L, Bressel HU, et al: Tamsulosin treatment of 19,365 patients with lower urinary tract symptoms: does co-morbidity alter tolerability? *J Urol* 1998;160(3 pt 1):784-791.

75. Lepor H, Williford WO, Barry MJ, et al: The efficacy of terazosin, finasteride, or both in benign prostatic hyperplasia. Veterans Affairs Cooperative Studies Benign Prostatic Hyperplasia Study Group. *N Engl J Med* 1996;335:533-539.

76. Bautista OM, Kusek JW, Nyberg LM, et al: Study design of the Medical Therapy of Prostatic Symptoms (MTOPS) trial. *Control Clin Trials* 2003;24:224-243.

77. McConnell JD, Roehrborn CG, Bautista OM, et al: The long-term effect of doxazosin, finasteride, and combination therapy on the clinical progression of benign prostatic hyperplasia. *N Engl J Med* 2003;349:2387-2398.

78. Siami P, Roehrborn CG, Barkin J, et al: Combination therapy with dutasteride and tamsulosin in men with moderate-to-severe benign prostatic hyperplasia and prostate enlargement: the CombAT (Combination of Avodart(R) and Tamsulosin) trial rationale and study design. *Contemp Clin Trials* 2007;28:770-799.

79. Keam SJ, Scott LJ: Dutasteride: a review of its use in the management of prostate disorders. *Drugs* 2008;68:463-485.

80. Roehrborn CG, Siami P, Barkin J, et al: The effects of dutasteride, tamsulosin and combination therapy on lower urinary tract symptoms in men with benign prostatic hyperplasia and prostatic enlargement: 2-year results from the CombAT study. *J Urol* 2008;179:616-621.

81. Kaplan SA, Roehrborn CG, Rovner ES, et al: Tolterodine and tamsulosin for treatment of men with lower urinary tract symptoms and overactive bladder: a randomized controlled trial. *JAMA* 2006;296:2319-2328.

82. McVary K: Lower urinary tract symptoms and sexual dysfunction: epidemiology and pathophysiology. *BJU Int* 2006;97 (suppl 2):23-28; discussion 44-45.

83. Kaminetsky JC: Comorbid LUTS and erectile dysfunction: optimizing their management. *Curr Med Res Opin* 2006;22: 2497-2506.

84. Gonzalez RR, Kaplan SA: Tadalafil for the treatment of lower urinary tract symptoms in men with benign prostatic hyperplasia. *Expert Opin Drug Metab Toxicol* 2006;2:609-617.

85. Sairam K, Kulinskaya E, McNicholas TA, et al: Sildenafil influences lower urinary tract symptoms. *BJU Int* 2002;90:836-839.

## Chapter 5

# Open Surgical and Endourologic Treatments

M edical pharmacotherapies have become the first-line treatments for men presenting with mild-to-moderate lower urinary tract symptoms (LUTS) (see Chapter 4 on medical therapies for benign prostatic hyperplasia [BPH]).[1] Although the long-term outcomes of these medical therapies have not yet been fully elucidated, the short-term measures appear to have efficacy in reducing the occurrence and progression of LUTS.[1,2] However, when choosing medical therapies, patients must understand the requirement to adhere to a strict, life-long medication schedule and should be prepared for the potential side effects of these medications. They must also be aware that the outcome indicators for these therapies may not be achieved as effectively or as reliably as with surgical intervention. Despite these inadequacies, however, patients may opt for medical therapy because of the perceived reduced risk of adverse events and the desire to avoid surgery.

Surgical treatment is an attractive alternative for patients who experience moderate-to-severe obstructive or irritative voiding symptoms, who have evidence of genitourinary complications (eg, renal compromise, bladder decompensation, recurrent urinary tract infections [UTIs], recurrent hematuria, bladder calculi), who have failed medical therapy, or who choose not to be managed medically. It has been shown that surgical treatments for BPH have long-term efficacy. Patients are often enthusiastic about surgical options if they are offered a one-time method to treat their LUTS, provided the method offers reduced risk and allows an efficacy equal to that of medical therapy.

The decision to initiate surgical treatment for BPH must take into account many factors including patient and physician preferences. Absolute indications for surgery include the presence of moderate-to-severe LUTS (American Urological Association Symptom Index [AUA-SI] ≥8), bladder calculi, renal failure due to bladder outlet obstruction (BOO), acute urinary retention (AUR), recurrent UTIs, and renal insufficiency. Once the decision for surgery has been made, then the size of the gland, patient comorbidities, and bladder comorbidities (eg, calculi, diverticula) should help guide which type of surgery should be performed. Medical therapy should be offered if a patient refuses surgical treatment. Figure 5-1 demonstrates the treatment algorithm that should be used when choosing a surgical option for the treatment of BPH.

Open prostatectomy was one of the first surgical procedures that attempted to definitively treat BPH. However, this procedure is relatively invasive and associated with comorbidities. In fact, open prostatectomy is now reserved for

---

**Figure 5-1:** Algorithm for choosing a surgical option to treat BPH. AUA-SI=American Urological Association Symptom Index; AUR=acute urinary retention; BOO=bladder outlet obstruction; DRE=digital rectal examination; HoLEP=holmium laser enucleation of the prostate; LUTS=lower urinary tract symptoms; MITs=minimally invasive treatments; PFS=pressure-flow study; PSA=prostate-specific antigen; QOL=quality of life; TUIP=transurethral incision of the prostate; TUMT=transurethral microwave thermotherapy; TUNA=transurethral needle ablation; TURP=transurethral resection of the prostate; TUVP=transurethral electrovaporization of the prostate; UTIs=urinary tract infections

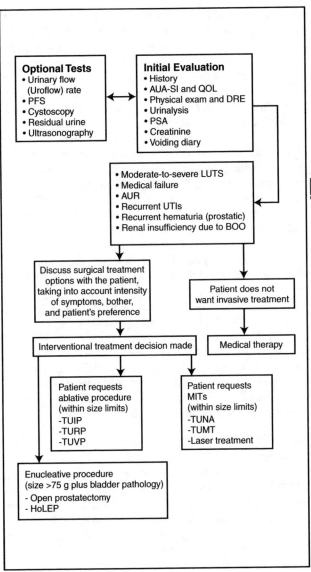

**Optional Tests**
- Urinary flow (Uroflow) rate
- PFS
- Cystoscopy
- Residual urine
- Ultrasonography

**Initial Evaluation**
- History
- AUA-SI and QOL
- Physical exam and DRE
- Urinalysis
- PSA
- Creatinine
- Voiding diary

- Moderate-to-severe LUTS
- Medical failure
- AUR
- Recurrent UTIs
- Recurrent hematuria (prostatic)
- Renal insufficiency due to BOO

Discuss surgical treatment options with the patient, taking into account intensity of symptoms, bother, and patient's preference

Patient does not want invasive treatment

Interventional treatment decision made

Medical therapy

Patient requests ablative procedure (within size limits)
-TUIP
-TURP
-TUVP

Patient requests MITs (within size limits)
-TUNA
-TUMT
-Laser treatment

Enucleative procedure (size >75 g plus bladder pathology)
- Open prostatectomy
- HoLEP

5

men presenting with symptomatic BPH and a large (>100 g) prostate with or without concomitant bladder pathologies (see below). In the 1930s, a less invasive procedure, transurethral resection of the prostate (TURP), replaced open prostatectomy as the 'gold standard' for the treatment of BPH.[3] However, TURP is still associated with significant morbidity and complications, including bleeding, transurethral resection (TUR) syndrome, incontinence, urethral strictures, retrograde ejaculation, and impotence.[4-7] These complications, coupled with high health-care costs associated with prolonged hospitalization, have sparked a movement to develop alternative endourologic procedures for the treatment of BPH that are durable, cost effective, and have fewer morbidities. In the past 20 years, additional endourologic treatments based on the technology of TURP have been developed as alternatives. To be preferred over open prostatectomy and TURP, these new minimally invasive treatments (MITs) must achieve significant subjective and objective success in most cases, have long-lasting results, and significantly reduce the morbidity historically associated with open surgery and TURP.

This chapter reviews the current surgical techniques used for the treatment of LUTS due to BPH. When choosing a therapy for a patient, it is important to understand the risks and benefits associated with each procedure and to assess the patient based on the severity of that patient's symptoms, his overall health status, and associated comorbidities.

## Open Prostatectomy

As mentioned above, TURP and the more modern MITs are the most common surgical procedures used to treat BPH in the United States today. However, many patients with markedly enlarged prostates (EPs) with or without concomitant bladder disorders, such as bladder diverticula or calculi, are often not amenable to this treatment option. For these patients, open prostatectomy continues to be a viable and preferred treatment option.[8]

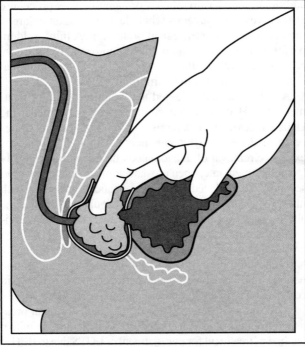

**Figure 5-2:** Schematic representation of the retropubic open prostatectomy. Modified from http://www.urolog.nl/urolog/images/menu/millin.jpg.

Currently, three methods of open enucleation of hyperplastic prostatic adenoma exist—retropubic, suprapubic, and perineal (percutaneous).[8] Retropubic open prostatectomy provides direct visualization of the adenomatous tissue with minimal surgical trauma to the bladder and precise transection of the urethra (Figure 5-2). Additionally, this approach is preferred for prostatic enlargement associated with prominent intraurethral components. Suprapubic gland enucleation is often considered when direct access to the bladder is required, most often in cases involving additional bladder diverticula or calculi.[8] This procedure also proves advantageous when dealing with an enlarged median lobe with intravesical protrusion. A third, seldom performed method is the perineal approach. The primary advantage of this method lies in the lack of an abdominal incision, most useful in the morbidly obese.

Although once considered the 'gold standard' for treatment of BPH, open prostatectomy is rarely performed in the United States today; it comprises <3% of surgical procedures performed for BPH management.[9] Although it provides extensive removal of adenomatous tissue with a relatively low retreatment rate, open prostatectomy is now rarely used secondary to a reduced prevalence of patients presenting with markedly enlarged prostate glands. Undoubtedly, this decline also reflects a general paradigm shift away from open surgical interventions toward medical therapies and MITs. Open prostatectomy has also been associated with relatively lengthy hospitalization periods (ie, 2 to 4 days), long recuperation periods, and perceived greater perioperative blood loss in comparison with contemporary alternative methods.[10]

A recent prospective series of the results of open prostatectomy indicated that it remains a viable and definitive method of treatment for management of LUTS due to BPH.[11] Specifically, 56 patients underwent open prostatectomy and received up to 11 years of postoperative follow-up. Mean intraoperative blood loss for these patients was 1,181.3 +/- 113.7 mL, with 36% of patients requiring a blood transfusion in the perioperative period. Two patients presented perioperatively with clot retention, three (5.4%) patients experienced subsequent urethral strictures, and three (5.4%) patients had bladder neck contractures. All patients experienced significant decreases in their AUA-SI and quality-of-life (QOL) scores. Less than 2% of patients required continued medication for symptomatic BPH after treatment.

Thus, open prostatectomy should still be considered for patients who present with large prostate glands, with or without concomitant bladder pathology, and who desire a definitive and effective long-term treatment. Although intra-operative blood loss can be a significant problem with this procedure, hemorrhage can be controlled intraoperatively and managed with autologous blood transfusion, if necessary. In fact, it should be recommended that all patients donate autologous blood before the procedure. However, results from long-term follow-up demonstrate lasting symptomatic improvement with this procedure, as well as a rare need for further medical therapy or surgical treatment.

## Transurethral Resection of the Prostate

Because it is less invasive than open prostatectomy, TURP has become the 'gold standard' for the treatment of patients with moderate-to-severe symptoms due to BPH.[3] By the 1990s, TURP far surpassed the frequency rate of open prostatectomy and accounted for >90% of the surgical procedures performed in the United States for the treatment of BPH.[3] Yet, many studies have indicated that the TURP procedure continues to be associated with many complications and comorbidities, including intraoperative bleeding, TUR syndrome, urethral stricture, bladder neck contracture, cardiovascular disorders, and perforation.[3,4,12-15] Within the past decade, improvements in operative techniques, video endoscopy, anesthetic care, and intraoperative monitoring of fluid and electrolytes have decreased the rates of morbidity and mortality associated with TURP.[16]

TURP is an endoscopic procedure (Figure 5-3) that requires general or spinal anesthesia and takes 30 to 60 minutes to perform. During the TURP procedure, the surgeon uses a resectoscope and a wire-loop electrode to remove obstructing prostatic tissue. Irrigating fluid is used throughout the procedure to maintain the surgeon's visibility and carry the resected pieces of tissue (chips) into the bladder, which are then flushed out at the end of the procedure.

TURP requires urethral catheterization for 24 to 48 hours, and a hospital stay ranging from 1 to 5 days (mean is 2 days).[17,18] Retrospective studies have suggested that

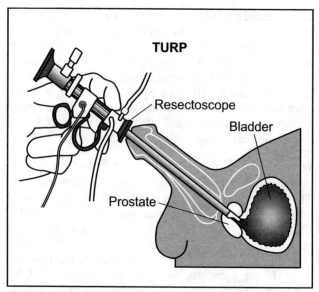

**Figure 5-3:** Schematic visualization of the TURP procedure. TURP=transurethral resection of the prostate

the overall rate of intraoperative complications associated with TURP is between 2% and 30%, averaging closer to 3%.[19,20] These immediate complications include a mortality rate significantly <0.2% caused by intraoperative myocardial infarction (MI) and cardiovascular compromise.[21] The most common intraoperative complication associated with TURP is bleeding, which requires transfusion in approximately 2% to 25% of patients.[17,22] It should be noted that the Veterans Affairs Cooperative (VA COOP) study, one of the largest and most comprehensive studies conducted on TURP to date, reported a transfusion rate of 4% to 5%, although the estimated national frequency is closer to 8%.[17,22]

A unique complication associated with the TURP procedure is TUR syndrome.[23] This syndrome is believed to result from the hyponatremia, hypervolemia, and hyperammonemia caused by the patient's metabolism if absorbed glycine is present in the nonconductive irrigative fluids used during TURP. TUR syndrome comprises a constellation of symptoms beginning intraoperatively and including hypotension, bradycardia, confusion, nausea, and vomiting. The incidence of TUR syndrome has not been definitely established, but ranges from 1% to 7% of patients undergoing the TURP procedure.[24] Recently, bipolar electrosurgical electrodes, compatible with saline instead of glycine, have been introduced to eliminate the occurrence of TUR syndrome.

The rate of retreatment (either medical or surgical) following TURP is as high as 20%.[25] In fact, recurring LUTS due to BPH requiring surgical intervention occurs in approximately 5% of patients over a 3-year period following TURP.[8,26] TURP is considered the 'gold standard' surgical treatment for BOO due to BPH, and it has been well studied. The reported intra-, peri-, and postoperative complications are listed in Table 5-1. The data presented are compiled from many different retrospective and prospective studies.[5,8,14-18,21,25-27]

TURP has been reported to cause some form of sexual dysfunction in many patients. For example, nearly 75% of men experience retrograde ejaculation and about 2% to 13% of men experience erectile dysfunction (ED) after TURP.[28] However, the numbers of new-onset ED must be evaluated objectively because ED is positively correlated with BPH progression and advancing age.[29,30] Therefore, many cases of ED reported after TURP may not have been because of the procedure itself but may be attributable to the natural effects of the aging process.

## Transurethral Electrovaporization of the Prostate

Alternative treatments have been developed that use similar endourologic principles as TURP but have also attempted to minimize comorbidities, such as significant

## Table 5-1: Reported Incidence of Complications Following TURP

**Intraoperative Complications (~3%)**

| | |
|---|---|
| Transurethral resection (TUR) syndrome | 1%-7% |
| Bleeding requiring transfusion | 8% |
| Deep-vein thrombosis (DVT) | 1%-2% |
| Pulmonary embolism | <1% |
| Urethral injury | 0%-2% |
| Bladder injury | 0%-2% |
| Mortality | <0.2% |

**Perioperative Complications**

| | |
|---|---|
| Persistent irritative voiding symptoms | 15%-25% |
| Clot retention | 3%-20% |
| Dysuria | 2%-16% |
| Urinary retention | 2%-8% |
| Transient hematuria | 4%-7% |
| Urinary tract infection (UTI) | 6%-20% |
| Transient incontinence | 1%-4% |
| Septicemia | 0%-5% |
| Epididymo-orchitis | 3%-5% |
| Proctitis | <1% |
| Bladder spasm | 1%-2% |
| Mortality | <0.5% |

bleeding. Transurethral electrovaporization of the prostate (TUVP) is a modification of existing transurethral technology and has been viewed as one of the most promising alternatives to TURP. The TUVP technique is a modification

**Long-term Complications**

| | |
|---|---|
| Retrograde ejaculation | 75%-85% |
| Erectile dysfunction (ED) | 2%-13% |
| Retreatment (TURP) | 3%-8% |
| Urinary incontinence | 1%-3% |
| Urethral stricture | 1%-2% |
| Bladder neck contracture | 1%-3% |
| Meatal stricture | ~1% |
| Chronic urinary tract infection (UTI) | ~1% |
| Chronic dysuria | <1% |
| Chronic urinary retention | <1% |
| Chronic prostatitis | <1% |
| Hematospermia | <1% |
| Hematuria | <1% |

5

of TURP in which obstructing prostatic tissue is vaporized instead of being removed in pieces. The TUVP procedure uses a grooved-roller electrode instead of the conventional loop used in TURP. This special electrode permits the simultaneous vaporization, desiccation, and coagulation of prostatic tissue using radiofrequency electrical current.[31] The advantage of TUVP over TURP is its association with little or no bleeding, fluid absorption, or electrolyte imbalance. In addition, TUVP has been shown to decrease the AUA-SI by about 60% to 85% and more than double the mean peak urinary flow rate ($Q_{max}$).[32-34] One prospective randomized control trial suggests that these effects are durable and associated with a relatively low recurrence of LUTS due to BPH.[35]

TUVP is not completely free from complications. For example, TUVP is still a transurethral procedure that requires general or spinal anesthesia and lasts for approximately 45 to 60 minutes. This potentially increases the likelihood of intraoperative myocardial events and other complications. Increased anesthesia requirements also necessitate a hospital stay, with an average postoperative hospital course of about 1 to 4 days.[32,36] Other intraoperative complications reported with TUVP include a 0% to 5% risk of prostatic capsule perforation or damage to bladder mucosa.[37] Because TUVP involves electrodesiccation of the prostatic tissue during the procedure, blood transfusions are rarely required, occur infrequently, and are not considered a substantial risk by the AUA (<1%).[38]

TUR syndrome can occur any time irrigation and glycine solutions are used during a procedure, and it has been reported during TUVP.[39] However, during TUVP, a zone of desiccation develops below the vaporized tissue that is believed to prohibit any dangerous irritant reabsorption and significantly minimize the occurrence of TUR syndrome.[31]

Peri- and postoperative complications occur in approximately 33% to 43% of patients undergoing TUVP.[32] By far the most common perioperative complication is irritative voiding symptoms, which occurs in 15% to 25% of patients within the first 1 to 2 weeks following TUVP.[40]

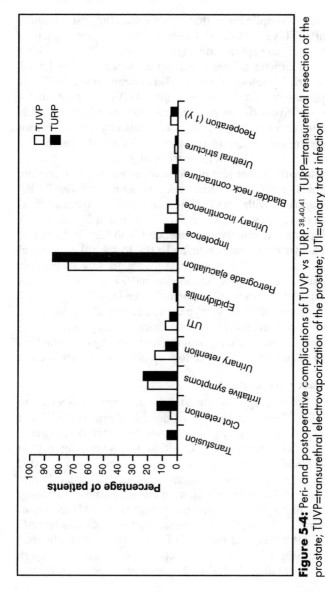

**Figure 5-4:** Peri and postoperative complications of TUVP vs TURP.[38,40,41] TURP=transurethral resection of the prostate; TUVP=transurethral electrovaporization of the prostate; UTI=urinary tract infection

Other complications that occur within the first 3 months after TUVP include AUR (6% to 23%), clot retention (0% to 5%), and epididymitis (0% to 1.4%).[32,35,42]

Treatment failure requiring a reoperation for LUTS or urinary retention due to BPH occurs in 4% to 7% of patients within the first year after TUVP.[38] A meta-analysis of five different prospective randomized control trials demonstrated this rate is not statistically different from the treatment failure reported for TURP (Figure 5-4).[40] In fact, the data from those trials suggest that there is a significantly higher rate of blood transfusion, clot retention, epididymitis, and bladder neck contracture following TURP compared with TUVP. However, postoperative complications reported following TUVP include a 3% to 18.6% incidence of urinary incontinence, 0% to 4.2% incidence of bladder neck contracture, and a 0% to 4% risk of urethral stricture.[32,34,38,40] Approximately 74% to 92% of patients experience retrograde ejaculation and 0% to 14% of patients report new-onset ED/impotence after TUVP.[32]

In summary, TUVP appears to be a promising alternative to TURP because TUVP has clinical efficacy and low morbidity. However, additional studies involving large numbers of patients and longer follow-up periods are warranted.

## Laser Treatments

Laser energy harvested for the treatment of BOO due to BPH offers a promising and durable alternative to TURP. Laser use in urology is not novel. Since the development of endoscopic lasers in the 1970s, the use of lasers within the field of urology has expanded immensely and included the treatment of symptomatic BPH. To date, four different types of lasers have been used for this purpose, including holmium:yttrium-aluminum-garnet (Ho:YAG), neodymium:YAG (Nd:YAG), potassium titanyl phosphate:YAG (KTP:YAG), and the diode laser.[43] The energy obtained from these lasers is delivered to the prostate tissue through different fibers including a right-angled fiber (side-firing),

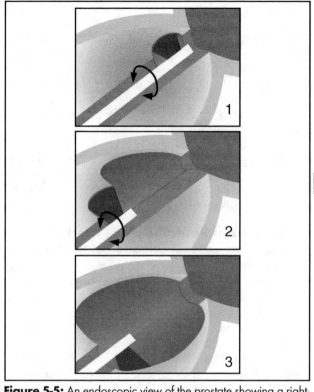

**Figure 5-5:** An endoscopic view of the prostate showing a right-angled fiber delivering laser energy to the prostate.

bare fiber (end-firing), contact tip fiber, or an interstitial fiber (Figure 5-5).[43]

Laser energy can be used to remove obstructing prostatic adenoma through tissue coagulation (at 60°C to 700°C), vaporization (>1,000°C), by excision of the tissue, or by a combination of these techniques. The extent to which the laser can cause either coagulation or vaporization is varied by adjusting the settings, including the power, wavelength, and exposure time settings.[44] The coagulation technique produces a necrosis deep within the prostatic tissue and results in a secondary tissue sloughing into the urethra for several weeks after treatment.[45] In contrast, laser-induced vaporization produces immediate tissue ablation at the surface of the prostate with a lesser degree of penetration and secondary tissue slough.[43] Both laser methods have been used to remove prostatic adenoma and have varying clinical efficacies. Overall, laser technologies are continuously evolving. By adjusting the extent to which the laser is used to coagulate or vaporize adenomatous tissue, or by adjusting the type of delivery fiber, urologists hope to discover the perfect laser technology, which would provide an efficacious, durable treatment for obstructing prostatic tissue, as well as minimize comorbidities.

## Holmium Laser Resection of the Prostate and Holmium Laser Enucleation of the Prostate

Holmium laser resection of the prostate (HoLRP) was popularized in 1994 when the relatively high-powered Ho:YAG laser became commercially available.[46,47] HoLRP uses the Ho:YAG laser for the incision, ablation, and resection of the prostate with the goal of relieving LUTS due to BPH with minimum loss of blood.

Technically, HoLRP uses a continuous flow resectoscope with a circular fiber guide in the tip of the scope. An end-firing laser fiber is used as the cutting instrument to precisely resect large pieces of prostatic tissue. Normal saline is used to dissipate thermal energy delivered by the holmium laser and, therefore, alleviate the risk of TUR syndrome (see above). The resected prostatic pieces are removed with a modified resectoscope loop.[48] The procedure minimizes blood loss because the holmium wavelength causes superficial coagulation (to a depth of 3 to 4 mm), producing adequate hemostasis for vessels up to 1 mm in diameter.[48,49] An additional benefit of HoLRP technology is that it can simultaneously be used for other endourologic applications (eg, to remove bladder calculi).

coagulate prostatic tissue. As with other coagulative lasers, the tissue eventually becomes necrotic and sloughs off during the weeks following the procedure and relieves bladder neck obstruction (BNO). VLAP uses a simple quartz laser fiber with a distal metallic reflecting mechanism to deflect the Nd: YAG laser beam at a right angle (side-firing) into the prostatic parenchyma. Although VLAP has been extensively studied, it has been difficult to summarize the statistical evidence because of inconsistent means used by investigators (eg, the number of treatments per patient, energy used, method of delivery) to evaluate this procedure.[38] A few trials have directly compared VLAP with TURP.[57-59] One multicenter randomized, controlled trial conducted in the United States at six investigational sites found that the AUA symptom score improved by 13.3 points in the TURP group and by 9 points in the VLAP group, and the $Q_{max}$ improved by 7 mL/sec in the TURP group and by 5.3 mL/sec in the VLAP group. Although the improvement in the AUA symptom score was statistically improved in patients who had TURP compared with VLAP, VLAP patients still reported an average of 78.2% improvement in their QOL score up to 1 year after undergoing the procedure.[57] However, other long-term studies suggest that VLAP may not have the durability of TURP[60]; but because of a lower morbidity rate, VLAP is still used, either by itself or in a hybrid technique with other treatments.

Similar to TURP, VLAP is usually performed under either general or spinal anesthesia. Despite this, it has been demonstrated that VLAP requires less operating time (23.4 vs 45.2 minutes) and a shorter hospitalization (1.8 vs 3.1 days) than TURP.[57] One reason for the decreased hospitalization time may be related to the fact that VLAP uses a coagulative technique, which minimizes blood loss. In fact, there have been almost no reports of blood transfusion after undergoing VLAP.[57,61] This relative lack of blood loss allows VLAP to be performed on patients who are either on full anticoagulation therapy or have abnormal coagulation indices because of hematologic disorders.[62]

| VLAP | ILC |
| --- | --- |
| <1% | <1% |
| <1% | <1% |
| NR | NR |
| NR | NR |
| | |
| 10%-100% | 15%-70% |
| 0%-16% | 80%-100% |
| 20%-30% | 15%-35% |
| 4%-15% | 5%-35% |
| 0%-5% | <1% |
| 2%-3% | 1%-5% |
| <1% | <1% |
| | |
| 27%-33% | 2%-15% |
| 3%-5% | 1%-2% |
| 5%-16% | 0%-15% |
| 0%-2% | 1%-5% |
| 1%-2% | NR |
| 4%-5% | <1% |

Perioperative complications after VLAP include clot retention (0% to 5%), hematuria (0% to 16%), epididymitis (2% to 3%), prostatitis (<1%), and transient urinary incontinence (1% to 2%) (Table 5-2).[63] However, one of the most common sequela after a VLAP procedure is irritative voiding symptoms secondary to prostatic coagulation. Perineal pain (1% to 4%), hesitancy (1% to 2%), and dribbling (1% to 2%) have also been reported.[57] Thus, it is recommended that urinary catheterization after VLAP should be implemented for up to 7 days postoperatively. Other complications are listed in Figure 5-4.

Long-term complications after VLAP include a urethral stricture rate from 0% to 1.8%, meatal stenosis rate from 1% to 2%, and a bladder neck contracture rate from 4% to 5% (Table 5-2).[57,63] New-onset ED has been reported in 3% to 5% of patients after VLAP. Once again, this may or may not be a direct consequence of the procedure because the onset of ED is confounded by age factors. The retrograde ejaculation rate varies from 27% to 33% and is thus less frequent in VLAP compared with TURP. The rate of surgical retreatment for recurrent LUTS or AUR is higher for VLAP compared with TURP. One study found that 38% of VLAP patients, compared with 16% of TURP patients, required further surgical treatment for BPH at 3 years.[60]

Recommendations have been made in an attempt to minimize comorbidities and lower the retreatment rate associated with VLAP. For example, it was found that patients with large prostates (ie, 80 to 100 g) are not good candidates for VLAP because they require multiple treatments to remove a sufficient amount of prostate tissue. In addition, patients with chronic UTI or bacterial prostatitis are also not considered ideal candidates because coagulated tissue may become infected. Overall, the VLAP technique is associated with a lower number of serious morbidities (ie, those requiring intervention) compared with TURP. However, the major disadvantage of VLAP compared with TURP is the relatively slow resolution of symptoms postoperatively and the extended need for urinary catheter drainage. Therefore, alternatives using vaporizing laser technologies with the Nd:YAG laser are now being investigated as alternatives.

## Interstitial Laser Coagulation

ILC for the treatment of symptomatic BPH was first described clinically by Muschter et al[64] in 1992. Since then, several variations of the procedure have been introduced for the treatment of BPH. Similar to other laser treatments, the goal of ILC is to achieve a marked volume reduction of obstructing prostatic tissue. Unlike other laser technologies, ILC generates coagulation necrosis inside the prostatic tissue rather than at its surface. To this end, ILC can be performed using the transurethral approach or the perineal approach.[65] The more common transurethral approach is performed with standard cystoscopy, a solid-state diode laser, and a special fiber-optic laser delivery system. Under direct visualization, the laser fiber is introduced directly into the prostate through a small incision in the prostatic urethra. The fiber can be introduced as deeply and as often as necessary to effectively coagulate any amount of tissue at any desired location.[65] Many studies have been published to suggest that ILC is associated with minimal morbidity and reasonable efficacy. However, the reported degree of urinary symptom relief, as well as the increase in $Q_{max}$ post-ILC, has varied considerably between studies. For example, the subjective improvement in AUA symptom scores after ILC ranges from 50% to 300% while the increase in $Q_{max}$ also spans from 5 to >10mL/sec.[64,66,67]

Intraoperative complications are rarely reported with ILC[66,68]; it is believed this is because of the relatively short operation time (ie, 30 to 60 minutes), as well as the fact that ILC can be performed under either local (eg, periprostatic block), regional (eg, spinal), or general anesthesia. The majority of patients (>90%) tolerate the procedure without any difficulty. Of those who experience discomfort during the procedure, orally administered pain medications can be used for relief. As with the laser technologies mentioned above, blood transfusion is not considered a risk associated with ILC because of the method of laser coagulation used. In addition, TUR syndrome and the lowering of serum sodium levels does not commonly occur with ILC (Table 5-2).[68]

In the perioperative period after ILC, irritative voiding symptoms are frequently reported and occur in up to 50% of patients (Table 5-2).[68] Occasionally, these symptoms will persist for up to 3 months.[69] In addition, many of these patients experience urinary retention due to the edema and inflammation from ILC. Therefore, postoperative urinary catheterization is often required for up to 1 month.[66,70] This catheterization period is significantly longer than for TURP,[71] and predisposes the patient to UTIs, which are present in as many as 35% of patients after ILC.[68] Other perioperative complications including prostatitis are listed in Figure 5-4.

Long-term complications arising from ILC include bladder neck contractures (<1%) and urethral strictures (1% to 5%) (Table 5-2). Other postoperative complications include new-onset ED (1% to 2%) and retrograde ejaculation (2% to 15%).[66,68] Unfortunately, few studies have addressed the long-term outcome of ILC because most reports are based on 12-month follow-up data. However, at 1 year of follow-up, the rate of surgical retreatment ranges from 0% to 15%.[68] One long-term study evaluating the success of ILC at 3 years found approximately 40% of patients required either medical therapy or surgical treatment for symptoms due to BPH.[72] Thus, although the durability of ILC does not rival TURP, the incidence of serious comorbidities appears to be significantly decreased.

## Conclusions

The past several decades have witnessed a dramatic change in urologic surgery for the treatment of BPH. Although a need for open prostatectomy continues to exist for a select population of patients (ie, those with large prostatic burdens with or without coexisting bladder pathologies), trends demonstrate that most patients do not desire such invasive surgery. Alternative endourologic procedures have been successful in offering durable results for the treatment of symptomatic BPH. However, these treatments have not been without associated comorbidities, including TUR syndrome, blood loss, hospitalization, irritative voiding symptoms, and a need for catheterization for up to 6 weeks postoperatively. As a result, other MITs (see Chapter 6) are being developed for the treatment of LUTS due to BPH.

## References

1.   Chapple CR: Pharmacological therapy of benign prostatic hyperplasia/lower urinary tract symptoms: an overview for the practising clinician. *BJU Int* 2004;94:738-744.

2.   Clifford GM, Farmer RD: Medical therapy for benign prostatic hyperplasia: a review of the literature. *Eur Urol* 2000;38:2-19.

3.   Bruskewitz RC, Christensen MM: Critical evaluation of transurethral resection and incision of the prostate. *Prostate Suppl* 1990;3:27-38.

4.   Doll HA, Black NA, McPherson K, et al: Mortality, morbidity and complications following transurethral resection of the prostate for benign prostatic hypertrophy. *J Urol* 1992;147:1566-1573.

5.   Horninger W, Unterlechner H, Strasser H, et al: Transurethral prostatectomy: mortality and morbidity. *Prostate* 1996;28:195-200.

6.   Mebust WK: Surgical management of benign prostatic obstruction. *Urology* 1988;32:12-15.

7.   Mebust WK, Holtgrewe HL, Cockett AT, et al: Transurethral prostatectomy: immediate and postoperative complications. A cooperative study of 13 participating institutions evaluating 3,885 patients. *J Urol* 1989;141:243-247.

8.   Grayhack JT, McVary KT, Kozlowski JM: *Benign Prostatic Hyperplasia*. Philadelphia, PA, Lippincott Williams & Wilkins, 2002, pp 1401-1470.

9.   Bruskewitz R: Management of symptomatic BPH in the US: who is treated and how? *Eur Urol* 1999;36(suppl 3):7-13.

10.  Miller EA, Ellis WJ: *Complications of Open Prostatectomy*, 3rd ed. Philadelphia, PA, WB Saunders Co, 2001, pp 399-403.

11.   Helfand B, Mouli S, Dedhia R, et al: Management of lower urinary tract symptoms secondary to benign prostatic hyperplasia with open prostatectomy: results of a contemporary series. *J Urol* 2006;176:2557-2561.

12.   Bruskewitz RC, Larsen EH, Madsen PO, et al: 3-year followup of urinary symptoms after transurethral resection of the prostate. *J Urol* 1986;136:613-615.

13.   Chilton CP, Morgan RJ, England HR, et al: A critical evaluation of the results of transurethral resection of the prostate. *Br J Urol* 1978;50:542-546.

14.   Meyhoff HH, Nordling J: Long term results of transurethral and transvesical prostatectomy. A randomized study. *Scand J Urol Nephrol* 1986;20:27-33.

15.   Varkarakis J, Bartsch G, Horninger W: Long-term morbidity and mortality of transurethral prostatectomy: a 10-year follow-up. *Prostate* 2004;58:248-251.

16.   Lu-Yao GL, Barry MJ, Chang CH, et al: Transurethral resection of the prostate among Medicare beneficiaries in the United States: time trends and outcomes. Prostate Patient Outcomes Research Team (PORT). *Urology* 1994;44:692-698;discussion 698-699.

17.   Mebust WK, Holtgrewe HL, Cockett AT, et al: Transurethral prostatectomy: immediate and postoperative complications. Cooperative study of 13 participating institutions evaluating 3,885 patients. *J Urol* 2002;167:5-9.

18.   Schatzl G, Madersbacher S, Lang T, et al: The early postoperative morbidity of transurethral resection of the prostate and of 4 minimally invasive treatment alternatives. *J Urol* 1997;158:105-110.

19.   Kuntz RM, Lehrich K, Ahyai S: Does perioperative outcome of transurethral holmium laser enucleation of the prostate depend on prostate size? *J Endourol* 2004;18:183-188.

20.   Tuhkanen K, Heino A, Aaltomaa S, et al: Long-term results of contact laser versus transurethral resection of the prostate in the treatment of benign prostatic hyperplasia with small or moderately enlarged prostates. *Scand J Urol Nephrol* 2003;37:487-493.

21.   Roos NP, Wennberg JE, Malenka DJ, et al: Mortality and reoperation after open and transurethral resection of the prostate for benign prostatic hyperplasia. *N Engl J Med* 1989;320:1120-1124.

5

22. Wasson JH, Reda DJ, Bruskewitz RC, et al: A comparison of transurethral surgery with watchful waiting for moderate symptoms of benign prostatic hyperplasia. The Veterans Affairs Cooperative Study Group on Transurethral Resection of the Prostate. *N Engl J Med* 1995;332:75-79.

23. Hahn RG: The transurethral resection syndrome. *Acta Anaesthesiol Scand* 1991;35:557.

24. Hahn RG: Transurethral resection syndrome from extravascular absorption of irrigating fluid. *Scand J Urol Nephrol* 1993;27:387.

25. Floratos DL, Kiemeney LA, Rossi C, et al: Long-term followup of randomized transurethral microwave thermotherapy versus transurethral prostatic resection study. *J Urol* 2001;165:1533-1538.

26. Iversen P, Madsen PO: Short-term cephalosporin prophylaxis in transurethral surgery. *Clin Ther* 1982;5(suppl A):58-66.

27. Malenka DJ, Roos N, Fisher ES, et al: Further study of the increased mortality following transurethral prostatectomy: a chart-based analysis. *J Urol* 1990;144:224-227.

28. Brookes ST, Donovan JL, Peters TJ, et al: Sexual dysfunction in men after treatment for lower urinary tract symptoms: evidence from randomised controlled trial. *BMJ* 2002;324:1059-1061.

29. Korenman SG: Epidemiology of erectile dysfunction. *Endocrine* 2004;23:87-91.

30. McVary KT, McKenna ME: The relationship between erectile dysfunction and lower urinary tract symptoms: epidemiological, clinical, and basic science evidence. *Curr Urol Rep* 2004;5:251-257.

31. Djavan B, Madersbacher S, Klingler HC, et al: Outcome analysis of minimally invasive treatments for benign prostatic hyperplasia. *Tech Urol* 1999;5:12-20.

32. Kaplan SA, Te AE: Transurethral electrovaporization of the prostate: a novel method for treating men with benign prostatic hyperplasia. *Urology* 1995;45:566-572.

33. Kupeli B, Yalcinkaya F, Topaloglu H, et al: Efficacy of transurethral electrovaporization of the prostate with respect to standard transurethral resection. *J Endourol* 1998;12:591-594.

34. McAllister WJ, Gilling PJ: Vaporization of the prostate. *Curr Opin Urol* 2004;14:31-34.

58.  Noble SM, Coast J, Brookes S, et al: Transurethral prostate resection, noncontact laser therapy or conservative management in men with symptoms of benign prostatic enlargement? An economic evaluation. *J Urol* 2002;168:2476-2482.

59.  Sengor F, Erdogan K, Tuzluoglu D, et al: Neodymium:YAG visual laser ablation of the prostate. *Eur Urol* 1996;29:446-449.

60.  McAllister WJ, Absalom MJ, Mir K, et al: Does endoscopic laser ablation of the prostate stand the test of time? Five-year results from a multicentre randomized controlled trial of endoscopic laser ablation against transurethral resection of the prostate. *BJU Int* 2000; 85:437-439.

61.  Anson K, Nawrocki J, Buckley J, et al: A multicenter, randomized, prospective study of endoscopic laser ablation versus transurethral resection of the prostate. *Urology* 1995;46:305-310.

62.  Kingston TE, Nonnenmacher AK, Crowe H, et al: Further evaluation of transurethral laser ablation of the prostate in patients treated with anticoagulant therapy. *Aust N Z J Surg* 1995;65:40-43.

63.  Wheelahan J, Scott NA, Cartmill R, et al: Minimally invasive laser techniques for prostatectomy: a systematic review. The ASERNIP-S review group. Australian Safety and Efficacy Register of New Interventional Procedures—Surgical. *BJU Int* 2000; 86:805-815.

64.  Muschter R, Hessel S, Hofstetter A, et al: [Interstitial laser coagulation of benign prostatic hyperplasia]. *Urologe A* 1993;32: 273-281.

65.  Muschter R, Hofstetter A: Technique and results of interstitial laser coagulation. *World J Urol* 1995;13:109-114.

66.  Muschter R, Hofstetter A: [Treatment of benign prostatic hyperplasia syndrome. 2: Interventional therapy]. *MMW Fortschr Med* 2000;142(3 suppl):161-169.

67.  Pypno W, Husiatynski W: Treatment of a benign prostatic hyperplasia by Nd:YAG laser - own experience. *Eur Urol* 2000;38: 194-198.

68.  Laguna MP, Alivizatos G, De La Rosette JJ: Interstitial laser coagulation treatment of benign prostatic hyperplasia: is it to be recommended? *J Endourol* 2003;17:595-600.

69.  Te AE, Malloy TR, Stein BS, et al: Photoselective vaporization of the prostate for the treatment of benign prostatic hyperplasia:

12-month results from the first United States multicenter prospective trial. *J Urol* 2004;172:1404-1408.

70.   Martenson AC, De La Rosette JJ: Interstitial laser coagulation in the treatment of benign prostatic hyperplasia using a diode laser system: results of an evolving technology. *Prostate Cancer Prostatic Dis* 1999;2:148-154.

71.   Lynch WJ, Williams JC: Interstitial laser coagulation technique: clinical research updates. *World J Urol* 2000;18(suppl 1):S14-S15.

72.   Floratos DL, Sonke GS, Francisca EA, et al: Long-term follow-up of laser treatment for lower urinary tract symptoms suggestive of bladder outlet obstruction. *Urology* 2000;56:604-609.

# Chapter 6

# Minimally Invasive Treatments

Transurethral resection of the prostate (TURP) is considered the most effective endoscopic surgical treatment for patients with benign prostatic hyperplasia (BPH). However, while the efficacy and durability of TURP have been proven over time, so have the associated comorbidities, such as bleeding requiring transfusion, transurethral resection (TUR) syndrome, and retrograde ejaculation. Therefore, newer surgical treatments of BPH have been aimed at providing one-time minimally invasive treatments (MITs) that are associated with fewer complications than occur with TURP. The new modalities for the treatment of BPH can be divided into two groups: true MITs that use the thermal effects of different sources of energy on the prostatic tissue, and treatments that encompass improvements in surgical endoscopic techniques.

## Transurethral Microwave Thermotherapy

One MIT is transurethral microwave thermotherapy (TUMT), which uses a device to apply heat to the prostatic tissue that causes necrosis and relief of bladder outlet obstruction (BOO). TUMT is based on the finding that normal prostate cells undergo necrosis when exposed to temperatures in excess of 45° C for 30 minutes.[1,2] Unfortunately, the urethral pain threshold is approximately 45° C. Therefore, low-energy TUMT (LE-TUMT) devices that in-

## Table 6-1: Common LE-TUMT and HE-TUMT Devices

**LE-TUMT Devices**

| Product | Description |
| --- | --- |
| TherMatrx® | 7-15 watts, no cooling |
| Prolieve™ | Lower wattage and a balloon |

**HE-TUMT Devices**

| Product | Description |
| --- | --- |
| Prostatron® | >60 watts with cooling system |
| Targis® | >60 watts with cooling system |
| CoreTherm™ | >60 watts, no cooling, intraprostatic temperature needle |

HE-TUMT=higher-energy TUMT; LE-TUMT=low-energy TUMT

corporate urethral cooling instrumentation were developed to allow for these elevated temperatures to destroy prostatic tissue. To further enhance outcomes, higher-energy TUMT (HE-TUMT) machines capable of achieving prostatic temperatures >70° C while maintaining low urethral temperatures were developed to cause thermoablation and thermocoagulation of prostatic tissue (Table 6-1).[3]

Both LE-TUMT and HE-TUMT demonstrate improvements in lower urinary tract symptoms (LUTS) due to BPH. Although it has been demonstrated that HE-TUMT is associated with greater improvements in urinary symptom scores compared with LE-TUMT, improvements between 30% and 86% have been reported with both forms of TUMT.[4] While statistically significant improvements of as much as 55% in peak urinary flow rate ($Q_{max}$) have been reported with HE-TUMT, its long-term improvements are still debatable.[2,5-7] Although the improvements in $Q_{max}$ following LE-TUMT or HE-TUMT have not reached those associated with TURP, significant improvements in urinary symptoms have been reported for long periods.[8] In addition, the retreatment rate for recurrent LUTS due to BPH during a 3-year follow-up period has been reported to be about 25%.[8] Another study reported that by 2 years after treatment with TUMT, 46.9% of patients were using medical therapy with an $\alpha$-adrenergic antagonist and 17.6% of patients elected for retreatment with TURP.[9] Overall, the long-term effectiveness in the relief of LUTS after treatment with TUMT is still unclear.

One of the major advantages of TUMT is that it can be performed in a single 1-hour session as an outpatient procedure without general or spinal anesthesia. Despite this alleviation of inpatient hospitalization, TUMT is still associated with comorbidities. Reports of complications vary and range from 0% to 38%, based on the study and the investigators's criteria for complications.[2,10]

As with TURP, the adverse events associated with TUMT can be divided into intra-, peri-, and postoperative complications. The most common intraoperative complication is pain during the procedure. Although TUMT is usually well tolerated by patients, most patients perceive a mild feeling of perineal warmth and a slight sensation of urinary urgency during the procedure. About 5% to 7% of patients report significant perineal discomfort during the procedure, which can be minimized with pain medication or momentary interruption of microwave emission.[8]

An intraoperative advantage of the TUMT procedure is the significantly decreased need for blood transfusions compared with TURP. For example, a meta-analysis study demonstrated a mean blood loss of about 300 mL after TURP compared with no blood loss after TUMT.[11] In addition, because of the nature of the procedure and the lack of glycine irrigation, TUR syndrome is not considered to be a risk with TUMT.

The TUMT device was designed so that the balloon portion of the device is seated at the bladder neck, with the active portion of the antenna positioned within the prostate (Figure 6-1). Ideally, cooling fluid circulating within the urethral catheter protects the urethra from overheating. However, improper positioning can place other nonprostatic tissues at risk for necrosis during TUMT. Recently, the risk of serious injuries from TUMT for BPH has been reported by the US Food and Drug Administration (FDA).[12] This report included a description of 10 instances of fistula formation and six instances of clinically significant tissue damage to the penis/urethra that have required colostomies, partial amputation of the penis, and/or other interventions.[13] In addition, minor bladder and urethral injuries or perforations have been reported in up to 5% of patients undergoing TUMT.[1,14]

Perioperative complications associated with TUMT have also been investigated. Compared with TURP, urinary retention occurs in a significantly increased number of patients after TUMT (15% to 30%).[15] Prolonged indwelling catheterization after TUMT, as well as persistent necrotic tissue within the prostatic fossa, is thought to increase the risk of urinary tract infections (UTIs) (about 10% to 15%). However, this is not significantly greater than the incidence of UTIs after TURP.[15] Postprocedure irritative voiding symptom rates increased almost twofold in patients undergoing TUMT compared with patients undergoing TURP.[15] Other perioperative complications include transient urinary incontinence (1% to 3%) and epididymo-orchitis (<1%) after TUMT.[16]

Overall, the relatively new technology TUMT appears to be associated with significantly lower postoperative frequencies of urinary incontinence, bladder neck contractures, and urethral strictures compared with TURP.[15,17-19] Stress or urge urinary incontinence also is an infrequent (≤1%) complication of TUMT.[8,20]

Because of the elderly population and the overlapping prevalence of BPH and erectile dysfunction (ED), it is

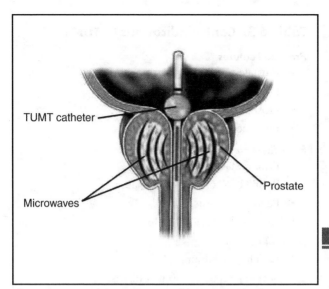

**Figure 6-1:** A schematic image of the transurethral microwave thermotherapy (TUMT) device. The balloon portion of the device is seated at the bladder neck, while the active portion of the antenna is positioned within the prostate.

difficult to demonstrate a causality between outcomes in MITs for BPH and changes in erectile function. Despite this difficulty, it has been reported that changes in sexual function occur in about 17% of men following TUMT compared with 36% following TURP.[21] One of the most common adverse effects after TUMT is retrograde ejaculation, which is reportedly observed in 48% to 90% of patients after TURP and between 0% to 28% of patients after TUMT.[21] Interestingly, it has been suggested that LE-TUMT protocols have a lower incidence of ED compared with HE-TUMT.[22,23]

Similar to TURP, there is an increased mortality rate associated with TUMT. For example, the risk of acute myocardial infarction (MI) is slightly increased follow-

## Table 6-2: Contraindications to TUMT

**Prostate Features**
- Prostate size <25 g
- Prostatic length <3 cm
- Prostate volume >100 g
- Prominent median lobe

**Prior Therapies**
- Prior radiation therapy
- Prior TURP or pelvic trauma
- Penile prosthesis
- Artificial urinary sphincter

**Medical History**
- Leriche's syndrome
- Severe peripheral vascular disease

TUMT=transurethral microwave thermotherapy;
TURP= transurethral resection of the prostate

---

ing TUMT. In a 3.9-year follow-up study of 888 patients undergoing TURP compared with 478 patients undergoing TUMT, both treatments had a higher incidence of acute MI, especially more than 2 years after therapy.[21] However, the mechanism of this is unknown.

The FDA has issued guidelines to minimize the risk of complications and appropriately select patients who would be ideal candidates for TUMT.[12] For example, it is important to ensure that the prostate gland is the eligible size indicated for the system being used (Table 6-2) so that thermotherapy is not applied to nonprostatic tissues. Prostates <25 g or a prostatic urethral length of <3 cm respond poorly to TUMT, as do patients with glands >100 g or patients with a prominent median bar. In addition, close attention should be paid to the placement of the urethral catheter and to rectal temperature sensors using acceptable methods (eg, direct visualization, ultrasound imaging), both before treatment and at other specified times consistent with manufacturer recommendations. In addition, to minimize the risk of rectal fistula formation, the patient should not have experienced prior radiation therapy in the pelvic area.

Other contraindications specific to TUMT are evolving as the technology changes and outcomes are studied more closely (Table 6-2). Patients with a history of TURP or pelvic trauma should not undergo TUMT because of potential alterations in pelvic anatomy. It also is now recommended that patients with penile prosthesis, severe urethral stricture disease, Leriche's syndrome, severe peripheral vascular disease, or an artificial urinary sphincter should avoid TUMT. Patients with pacemakers and defibrillators need clearance from their cardiologists before turning off their pacemakers during therapy.[14]

## Transurethral Needle Ablation of the Prostate

Another technique approved for treating patients with symptoms of BPH uses high-frequency radio waves to cause thermal injury to the prostate. Transurethral needle ablation (TUNA) of the prostate is a relatively new procedure that uses needles to deliver interstitial, low-level radio-frequency energy to produce a temperature above $100^\circ$ C and subsequently cause prostatic tissue necrosis (Figure 6-2).[24] The procedure duration averages 30 to 45 minutes.

Improvement in LUTS and resolution of BOO after TUNA is believed to occur because of reabsorption of the necrotic prostatic tissue and subsequent scar formation. Some studies have suggested that $\alpha$-adrenergic blockade may also contribute to improvement in LUTS from the necrosis of nerves within the prostate after TUNA.[25] Clinically, TUNA has been associated with about a 50% decrease in American Urological Association-International

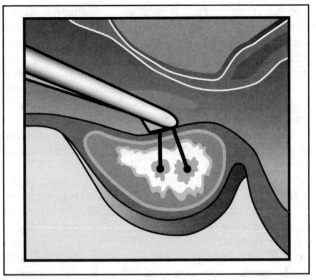

**Figure 6-2:** Schematic view of the transurethral needle ablation (TUNA) of the prostate procedure, in which the TUNA device is inserted intraurethrally. Needles deploy and engage prostatic tissue, and then radio-frequency energy is applied to create prostatic necrosis.

Prostate Symptom Scores (AUA-IPSS) and about a 70% improvement in $Q_{max}$.[26] As with TUMT, the long-term efficacy of TUNA remains to be determined. Compared with other treatments for symptomatic BPH, TUNA appears to be more effective than medical therapy, but less effective and durable than TURP in the treatment of BPH.[15] However, the complication rates after undergoing TUNA are significantly lower compared with TURP, which may be a trade-off between the procedures.

TUNA can be performed under local anesthesia, intravenous (IV) sedation, or transperineal prostate block. Therefore, TUNA does not require an additional hospital stay and is generally performed as an outpatient procedure that lasts

<30 minutes.[27] The most common intraoperative complication reported in TUNA is a burning sensation, which can be significant enough to cause the termination of the procedure in about 1% of patients.[28] However, this can be managed by a prostatic nerve block before beginning the procedure. Similar to many of the other MITs, TUNA avoids significant intraoperative bleeding by heat coagulation.[29]

The overall incidence of peri- and postoperative complications following TUNA is about 25% (Table 6-3), a rate that is significantly lower than with TURP.[29] Almost all patients undergoing TUNA are discharged and sent home with an indwelling catheter for 2 to 3 days.[15] In addition, most patients should be informed that they will experience mild dysuria for 1 to 2 weeks and mild hematuria for the first 2 to 3 days after the procedure.[26] The peri- and postoperative complications of TUNA are listed in Table 6-3.[26,30-32]

It should be stated that treatment failure, because of recurring LUTS due to BPH, has been reported in up to 25% of patients within 3 years and in up to 30% within 5 years after treatment.[13,15,33] Sexual and erectile dysfunction (ED) have also been evaluated postoperatively in patients after TUNA. Unlike TURP, retrograde ejaculation is a rare complication of TUNA, occurring in <1% of patients.[13,26]

The ideal patient for TUNA is a man who has obstructive BPH, a prostate of ≤100 g, and predominately lateral lobe enlargement.[15] Therefore, it is recommended that patients undergo a pre-TUNA cystoscopy and transrectal ultrasound to determine prostate anatomy. It should be stated that the presence of an enlarged median lobe is not a contraindication to TUNA. However, aggressive therapy to the bladder neck may theoretically increase the risk of retrograde ejaculation.[26]

## Prostatic Stents

The use of prostatic endoprostheses to maintain luminal patency is a well-established concept in various

## Table 6-3: Reported Incidence of Complications After TUNA

**Intraoperative Complications**

| | |
|---|---|
| Urethral burning sensation | 50%-100% |
| Severe pain requiring discontinuation of procedure | <1% |
| Urethral injury | 0% |
| Bladder injury | 0% |

**Perioperative Complications**

| | |
|---|---|
| Irritative voiding symptoms | 55%-100% |
| Perineal pain | ~50% |
| Urinary retention | 10%-40% |
| Urinary tract infection (UTI) | 8%-14% |
| Dysuria | 6%-7% |
| Epididymo-orchitis | 1%-5% |
| Clot retention | 1%-2% |
| Prostatitis | 1%-2% |
| Deep-vein thrombosis (DVT) | <2% |

surgical settings. Therefore, it is not unusual when this therapy is applied to the treatment of BOO due to BPH. Prostatic stents are designed as permanent and temporary devices (Figure 6-3). The major characteristic of permanent prostatic endoprostheses is that they allow tissue ingrowth that results in the stent becoming embedded in the urethral wall. Temporary stents are made of nonabsorbable material that retards epithelialization, which facilitates removal. As with many of the MITs, the data

**Long-term Complications**

| | |
|---|---|
| Retrograde ejaculation | <1% |
| Erectile dysfunction (ED) | 1%-3% |
| Retreatment (TURP) | 5% |
| Urinary incontinence | 1%-3% |
| Urethral stricture | 1%-2% |
| Bladder neck contracture | 1%-5% |
| Chronic prostatitis | <1% |
| Urinary incontinence | <1% |
| Retreatment | 20%-30% |

TUNA is a minimally invasive treatment (MIT) with a relatively low complication rate. The reported adverse events were obtained from the results of many retrospective and prospective studies.[13,15,24-28,33,34,37]

TUNA=transurethral needle ablation of the prostate; TURP= transurethral resection of the prostate

6

appear to be variable based on the type of stent used and the duration of the stent. For example, the improvement in IPSS is about 60% initially, but in some studies it can decrease to about 30% by 2 years.[35,36] Quality-of-life (QOL) scores remain significantly improved throughout most study periods, unless complications arise. One study using temporary stents reported that the $Q_{max}$ increased by 5.5 mL/sec 1 month postoperatively but returned to baseline by 3 months.[36] Therefore, while promising, the

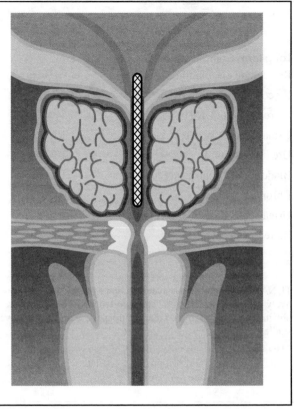

**Figure 6-3:** Schematic image of a prostatic stent, which can be temporary or permanent, depending on its material consistency and indwelling duration.

clinical efficacy of these stents still remains controversial for the treatment of BOO due to BPH.

There are now at least three different indications for the use of prostatic endoprostheses: permanent relief of BOO, transient relief of BOO, and diagnostic purposes. Prostatic stents were developed as an alternative MIT to provide permanent relief of prostatic obstruction. To date, permanent stents are used in elderly men with significant comorbidities who are therefore unfit for surgery.[38] This recommendation is based on a number of studies. For example, Perry et al[35] inserted a thermo-expandable stent in 211 men (average age 80 years) who were deemed unfit for surgery. During their 8-year follow-up, 38% of patients had died with their stents in place, 34% remained alive with their stents in place and functional, 23% had had their stents removed for failure, and 4% had had their stents removed because the stents were no longer required. Therefore, the long-term failure rate in this rather large series was about 25%. A recent study investigated whether stents should be used electively for the treatment of symptomatic BPH in elderly men. The results of this study overwhelmingly concluded that stents should not be used electively because only 37% of the stents remained in situ by 6 months and 78% were removed within 2 years after placement. In addition, about 20% of patients reported inter-mittent episodes of urge incontinence, 19% noticed transient hematuria, 17% reported retrograde ejaculation, and 6% had painful ejaculation. Another problem with permanent stents is that encrustation, UTI, chronic pain, and calculi forma-tion occur in 20% to 30% of these patients.[38] If endoscopic instrumentation becomes necessary, for instance, because of a bladder tumor, the stent usually must be removed to enable the insertion of a resectoscope. Therefore, when these issues are taken together, the conclusion is that permanent stents should be used only in high-risk patients who present with recurrent urinary retention (as an alternative to catheteriza-tion) and who are unfit for surgery.[37]

Stents have also been used to as temporary solutions to provide short-term relief of BOO after procedures such as interstitial laser coagulation (ILC), visual laser ablation of the prostate (VLAP), and HE-TUMT. In these proce-dures, temporary BOO can occur because of postoperative prostatic edema. Temporary stents have been used in this setting to relieve BOO, as well as to avoid the need for intermittent catheterization. All studies on this issue provide encouraging data that suggest that stents are useful in relieving temporary obstruction.[39-41]

For diagnostic purposes, prostatic stents have also been used to predict the outcome of TURP in difficult cases, such as those with a combination of BOO due to BPH and severe detrusor overactivity. For example, stents have been used to evaluate the results of TURP in patients suffering from neurologic conditions such as Parkinson's disease or multiple sclerosis. One such study evaluated 37 patients with prostatic stents and was able to predict who would respond well to TURP.[42]

Overall, prostatic stents offer potential therapies to a select group of patients who suffer from symptoms due to BOO. According to treatment guidelines, stents should be offered only as an alternative to permanent or intermittent catheterization in men who are unfit for invasive treatment. However, their use as a temporary relief of symptoms or as a diagnostic tool appears promising.

## Water-induced Thermotherapy

With the aging male population, there has been a relentless search to develop a durable treatment associated with few morbidities for the treatment of symptomatic BPH. One of the MITs that has recently emerged as a treatment alternative to TURP is water-induced thermotherapy (WIT). The goal of WIT is to produce heat-induced coagulative necrosis and secondary ablation of the prostatic adenoma.[43] The thermal energy used in WIT is derived from heated water that is circulated in a closed-loop system within a specially designed catheter. The catheter incorporates a balloon that is expanded during the procedure to increase the surface area in contact with the targeted tissue, ensuring uniform heat application and deep thermal penetration. WIT is an emerging technology, and there have been few studies to evaluate its efficacy and morbidities. However, initial studies performed in Europe suggest that

WIT has some clinical efficacy in reducing the frequency of LUTS as well as increasing $Q_{max}$.[44,45]

One of the major advantages promised by the WIT procedure is the alleviation of systemic analgesia or sedation. Topical lidocaine jelly (2%) is believed to provide sufficient analgesia.[44,45] Patients often report a sensation of moderate burning accompanied by urgency during the procedure. However, these symptoms are transient and disappear without intervention or stopping the procedure.[44]

Adverse outcomes following WIT are similar to the other MITs. These complications include epididymitis (3% to 4%), hematuria (20% to 25%), transient impotence (1% to 2%), transient urge incontinence (2% to 3%), UTI (30% to 35%), urethral pain (4% to 5%), and proctitis (<1%). Acute urinary retention (AUR) requiring recatheterization occurs in 10% to 15% of patients after WIT.[46] WIT shares the disadvantages of most other thermal-based, minimally invasive techniques in that postprocedural catheterization is required for the high incidence of dysuria and irritative voiding symptoms (11% to 12%) that occur because of tissue sloughing, edema, and inflammation.

A few studies suggest that WIT requires a secondary treatment in 5% to 6% of patients at 1 year.[46] However, additional clinical studies are needed to evaluate the durability and future potential of WIT.

## Conclusions

MITs are becoming popular alternative treatments to TURP for the treatment of BPH. These new, less invasive treatments use a variety of thermal-based treatments as well as new variations on older surgical techniques. The goals of these alternative treatments should include outcomes in which cost-effective benefits outweigh potential side effects that are acceptable to the patients.

Importantly, the less invasive treatments for BPH do not necessarily aim to achieve results similar to TURP. This is a trade-off for their decreased incidence of side effects and adverse outcomes. Thus, there is a fine balance between clinical efficacy and comorbidities. Less invasive procedures offer a wide range of clinical improvements but also entail unique complication profiles. The choice to use thermal-based MITs should involve an active discussion between the urologist and the patient, and should take into account patient preference, patient comorbidities, and the need for either a permanent solution (ie, open prostatectomy, TURP) or a temporary measure (ie, TUNA, TUMT) that may have to be repeated at regular intervals.

## References

1. Larson TR, Collins JM, Corica A: Detailed interstitial temperature mapping during treatment with a novel transurethral microwave thermoablation system in patients with benign prostatic hyperplasia. *J Urol* 1998;159:258-264.

2. Rubeinstein JN, McVary KT: Transurethral microwave thermotherapy for benign prostatic hyperplasia. *Int Braz J Urol* 2003; 9:251.

3. Brehmer M, Baba S: Transurethral microwave thermotherapy: how does it work? *J Endourol* 2000;14:611-615.

4. Thalmann GN, Mattei A, Treuthardt C, et al: Transurethral microwave therapy in 200 patients with a minimum follow-up of 2 years: urodynamic and clinical results. *J Urol* 2002;167:2496-2501.

5. d'Ancona FC, Francisca EA, Debruyne, FM, et al: High-energy transurethral microwave thermotherapy in men with lower urinary tract symptoms. *J Endourol* 1997;11:285-289.

6. Larson TR, Blute ML, Bruskewitz RC, et al: A high-efficiency microwave thermoablation system for the treatment of benign prostatic hyperplasia: results of a randomized, sham-controlled, prospective, double-blind, multicenter clinical trial. *Urology* 1998;51:731-742.

7. de la Rosette JJ, Francisca EA, Kortmann BB, et al: Clinical efficacy of a new 30-min algorithm for transurethral microwave thermotherapy: initial results. *BJU Int* 2000;86:47-51.

8. de la Rosette JJ, Laguna P, Gravas S, et al: Transurethral microwave thermotherapy: the gold standard for minimally invasive therapies for patients with benign prostatic hyperplasia? *J Endourol* 2003;17:245-251.

9.   Hallin A, Berlin T: Transurethral microwave thermotherapy for benign prostatic hyperplasia: clinical outcome after 4 years. *J Urol* 1998;159:459-464.

10.   Ohigashi T, Baba S, Ohki T, et al: Long-term effects of transurethral microwave thermotherapy. *Int J Urol* 2002;9:141-145.

11.   Wheelahan J, Scott NA, Cartmill R, et al: Minimally invasive non-laser thermal techniques for prostatectomy: a systematic review. The ASERNIP-S review group. *BJU Int* 2000;86:977-988.

12.   US Food and Drug Administration: FDA Public Health Notification: Serious injuries from microwave thermotherapy for benign prostatic hyperplasia. October 11, 2000. Available online at: http://www.fda.gov/cdrh/safety/bph.html. Accessed July 6, 2007.

13.   Tunuguntla HS, Evans CP: Minimally invasive therapies for benign prostatic hyperplasia. *World J Urol* 2002;20:197-206.

14.   Floratos DL, Sonke GS, Francisca EA, et al: High-energy transurethral microwave thermotherapy for the treatment of patients in urinary retention. *J Urol* 2000;163:1457-1460.

15.   AUA Practice Guidelines Committee: AUA guideline on the management of benign prostatic hyperplasia (2003), Chapter 1: Diagnosis and treatment recommendations. *J Urol* 2003;170:530-547.

16.   Terada N, Aoki, Y, Ichioka K, et al: Microwave thermotherapy for benign prostatic hyperplasia with the Dornier Urowave: response durability and variables potentially predicting response. *Urology* 2001;57:701-705; discussion 705-706.

17.   Dahlstrand C, Walden M, Geirsson G, et al: Transurethral microwave thermotherapy versus transurethral resection for symptomatic benign prostatic obstruction: a prospective randomized study with a 2-year follow-up. *Br J Urol* 1995;76:614-618.

18.   D'Ancona FC, Francisca EA, Witjes WP, et al: High-energy thermotherapy versus transurethral resection in the treatment of benign prostatic hyperplasia: results of a prospective randomized study with 1 year of follow-up. *J Urol* 1997;158:120-125.

19.   Floratos DL, Kiemeney LA, Rossi C, et al: Long-term follow-up of randomized transurethral microwave thermotherapy versus transurethral prostatic resection study. *J Urol* 2001;165:1533-1538.

20.   de la Rosette JJ, D'Ancona FC, Debruyne FM: Current status of thermotherapy of the prostate. *J Urol* 1997;157:430-438.

21.  Rubenstein J, McVary KT: E-medicine: Transurethral thermotherapy of the prostate. Available at: http://www.emedicine.com/med/topic3070.htm. Accessed July 6, 2007.

22.  Arai Y, Fukuzawa, S, Terai A, et al: Transurethral microwave thermotherapy for benign prostatic hyperplasia: relation between clinical response and prostate histology. *Prostate* 1996;28:84-88.

23.  Francisca EA, d'Ancona FC, Hendriks JC, et al: Quality of life assessment in patients treated with lower energy thermotherapy (Prostasoft 2.0): results of a randomized transurethral microwave thermotherapy versus sham study. *J Urol* 1997;158:1839-1844.

24.  Chapple CR, Issa MM, Woo H: Transurethral needle ablation (TUNA). A critical review of radiofrequency thermal therapy in the management of benign prostatic hyperplasia. *Eur Urol* 1999;35: 119-128.

25.  Rasor JS, Zlotta AR, Edwards SD, et al: Transurethral needle ablation (TUNA): thermal gradient mapping and comparison of lesion size in a tissue model and in patients with benign prostatic hyperplasia. *Eur Urol* 1993;24:411-414.

26.  Roehrborn CG, Issa MM, Bruskewitz RC, et al: Transurethral needle ablation for benign prostatic hyperplasia: 12-month results of a prospective, multicenter U.S. study. *Urology* 1998;51:415-421.

27.  Ramon J, Lynch TH, Eardley I, et al: Transurethral needle ablation of the prostate for the treatment of benign prostatic hyperplasia: a collaborative multicentre study. *Br J Urol* 1997;80:128-134; discussion 134-135.

28.  Campo B, Bergamaschi F, Corrada P, et al: Transurethral needle ablation (TUNA) of the prostate: a clinical and urodynamic evaluation. *Urology* 1997;49:847-850.

29.  Schatzl G, Madersbacher S, Djavan B, et al: Two-year results of transurethral resection of the prostate versus four 'less invasive' treatment options. *Eur Urol* 2000;37:695-701.

30.  Braun M, Mathers M, Bondarenko B, et al: Treatment of benign prostatic hyperplasia through transurethral needle ablation (TUNA). Review of the literature and six years of clinical experience. *Urol Int* 2004;72:32-39.

31.  Daehlin L, Gustavsen A, Nilsen AH, et al: Transurethral needle ablation for treatment of lower urinary tract symptoms associated with benign prostatic hyperplasia: outcome after 1 year. *J Endourol* 2002;16:111-115.

32. Rosario DJ, Woo H, Potts KL, et al: Safety and efficacy of transurethral needle ablation of the prostate for symptomatic outlet obstruction. *Br J Urol* 1997;80:579-586.

33. Zlotta AR, Giannakopoulos X, Maehlum O, et al: Long-term evaluation of transurethral needle ablation of the prostate (TUNA) for treatment of symptomatic benign prostatic hyperplasia: clinical outcome up to five years from three centers. *Eur Urol* 2003;44:89-93.

34. Bruskewitz R: Management of symptomatic BPH in the US: who is treated and how? *Eur Urol* 1999;36(suppl 3):7-13.

35. Perry MJ, Roodhouse AJ, Gidlow AB, et al: Thermo-expandable intraprostatic stents in bladder outlet obstruction: an 8-year study. *BJU Int* 2002;90:216-223.

36. van Dijk MM, Mochtar CA, Wijkstra H, et al: The bell-shaped nitinol prostatic stent in the treatment of lower urinary tract symptoms: experience in 108 patients. *Eur Urol* 2006;49:353-359.

37. Madersbacher S, Alivizatos G, Nordling J, et al: EAU 2004 guidelines on assessment, therapy and follow-up of men with lower urinary tract symptoms suggestive of benign prostatic obstruction (BPH guidelines). *Eur Urol* 2004;46:547-554.

38. Ogiste JS, Cooper K, Kaplan SA: Are stents still a useful therapy for benign prostatic hyperplasia? *Curr Opin Urol* 2003;13:51-57.

39. Laaksovirta S, Isotalo T, Talja M, et al: Interstitial laser coagulation and biodegradable self-expandable, self-reinforced poly-L-lactic and poly-L-glycolic copolymer spiral stent in the treatment of benign prostatic enlargement. *J Endourol* 2002;16:311-315.

40. Petas A, Isotalo T, Talja M, et al: A randomised study to evaluate the efficacy of a biodegradable stent in the prevention of postoperative urinary retention after interstitial laser coagulation of the prostate. *Scand J Urol Nephrol* 2000;34:262-266.

41. Petas A, Talja M, Tammela TL, et al: The biodegradable self-reinforced poly-DL-lactic acid spiral stent compared with a suprapubic catheter in the treatment of post-operative urinary retention after visual laser ablation of the prostate. *Br J Urol* 1997;80:439-443.

42. Knutson T: Can prostate stents be used to predict the outcome of transurethral resection of the prostate in the difficult cases? *Curr Opin Urol* 2004;14:35-39.

43. Corica FA, Cheng L, Ramnani D, et al: Transurethral hot-water balloon thermoablation for benign prostatic hyperplasia: patient tolerance and pathologic findings. *Urology* 2000;56:76-80.

6

44. Cioanta I, Muschter R: Water-induced thermotherapy for benign prostatic hyperplasia. *Tech Urol* 2000;6:294-299.

45. Muschter R, Schorsch I, Danielli L, et al: Transurethral water-induced thermotherapy for the treatment of benign prostatic hyperplasia: a prospective multicenter clinical trial. *J Urol* 2000;164:1565-1569.

46. Muschter R: Conductive heat: hot water-induced thermotherapy for ablation of prostatic tissue. *J Endourol* 2003;17:609-616.

# Chapter 7

# Complications of Open Surgery for BPH and LUTS

An excellent way to avoid complications from surgery is to use invasive options only when absolutely necessary. By following the accepted criteria for the intervention of bladder neck obstruction (BNO) caused by benign prostatic hyperplasia (BPH), both the urologist and the patient can frequently avoid trouble.

Acute urinary retention (AUR) often indicates end-stage bladder decompensation, which requires surgery. An attempt at decatheterization for patients presenting with an incident-related (eg, postoperative or acute bacterial prostatitis) or spontaneous episode of retention is reasonable. Using α-adrenergic antagonists in conjunction with this voiding trial is also worthwhile. For repeated episodes of retention, management by intermittent catheterization or continued catheter drainage is possible, but this is usually an unacceptable alternative to surgery.

Bilateral hydronephrosis with renal functional impairment requires the relief of the obstruction to preserve the integrity of the upper tracts. Once the catheter is inserted, postobstructive diuresis may occur, requiring meticulous fluid and electrolyte management. The patient's general condition should be optimized before undertaking surgical intervention.

Bladder decompensation often presents when there are multiple bladder calculi, prominent narrow-necked bladder diverticula, overflow incontinence, and other signs of end-stage bladder decompensation, which are indications for treatment. Recurrent or chronic urinary tract infections (UTIs) caused by elevated postvoid residual urine (PVR) are also an indication for considering intervention. Acute or chronic bacterial prostatitis should be excluded as a possible source of infection. A detailed patient history, physical examination, and lower tract localization cultures should help to clarify this issue.

Gross hematuria is an infrequent, but legitimate, indication for prostatectomy, particularly with multiple episodes and when associated with clot retention or significant blood loss. The usual limited initial hematuria associated with BPH should be managed conservatively. Antiandrogen measures, such as the use of 5α-reductase inhibitors (5ARIs) such as finasteride (Proscar®) and dutasteride (Avodart®) almost always have a favorable effect on recurrent prostatic bleeding.[1]

Obstructive and irritative voiding symptoms are common indications that lead to consideration of prostatic surgery and other therapeutic approaches. The cause of the symptoms should be established with a high degree of probability. Both the urologist and the patient must be clearly aware of the expected results and the risks involved in achieving those results.

Current evidence indicates that medical therapies have variable limited effectiveness in altering the symptoms and pathophysiologic effects of BPH. Use of drugs with established physiologic effects on the prostate or bladder, alone or combined, is reasonable in patients with acute or chronic voiding problems caused by BPH. But physicians should remember that prolonged exposure to therapies with limited effectiveness carries the risk of converting a reversible voiding dysfunction into a permanent one. Additionally, the least cost-effective use of health-care expenditure is serial treatment with multiple medications followed by surgical or minimally invasive treatments (MITs). Prioritizing these issues for and with patients remains a challenge for the urologist.

## Surgical Treatment

The goals of surgical treatment for BPH-related voiding dysfunction are to correct the significant physiologic effects of BNO and to improve the patient's quality of life (QOL); these are achieved when he is able to void to completion at normal intervals with an excellent urinary stream while retaining good urinary control and unaltered sexual function. The chosen treatment approach should allow these patient-prioritized goals to be reached with the least risk of morbidity and disability. The patient's general condition, size and configuration of the obstructing prostatic tissue, functional status of the bladder, the surgeon's skill, and the patient's preference warrant careful consideration if a prostatectomy is planned.

### Preoperative Preparation

Careful assessment of the patient's general and genitourinary status is essential to establish a proper diagnosis, to plan appropriate treatment, and to avoid complications. Prostatectomy is an elective procedure. Even in the patient with the most severe degree of BNO and its anatomic sequelae, an obstruction can be adequately relieved by catheter drainage while the patient's condition is optimized before definitive treatment. Adoption of this concept has played a major role in reducing the mortality and morbidity associated with surgical treatment of BPH.

### Systemic Considerations

The aged patient with BPH often has cardiovascular, pulmonary, neurologic, or other abnormalities that affect the choice of and preparation for a therapeutic approach, as well as the anesthetic used. Patients with chronic obstructive pulmonary disease (COPD), valvular heart disease, or ischemic heart disease may require sophisticated evaluation to provide baseline information, to focus preoperative management, and to help select the optimal anesthetic approach. Drug allergies and use of particular drugs (ie, aspirin or anti-inflammatory agents) that affect coagulation should be noted. The risks of postoperative deep-vein thrombosis (DVT) and pulmonary emboli also deserve special attention.

### Genitourinary Considerations

Renal failure resulting from BNO due to BPH is often reversible, although this is unpredictable. Catheter drainage of the bladder usually relieves the obstruction and results in maximum renal function improvement. Renal function status significantly affects appropriate anesthetic and pharmacologic management in these patients.

Sepsis has been a major contributor to infrequent mortality after prostate surgery.[2] Bacteremia occurs postoperatively in 10% to 32% of patients without recognized preoperative bacteriuria[3] and much more frequently in patients with infected urine.[4] Appropriately timed initiation of antibiotic therapy selected on the basis of in vitro culture findings is an accepted practice. Patients with increased risk factors for infection (ie, azotemia, upper tract calculi, significant PVR, debility, immunocompromised states, diabetes mellitus) are maintained on longer-term oral antibiotic prophylaxis.

## Open Prostatectomy and Suprapubic Prostatectomy

Factors influencing the choice of the suprapubic approach for enucleation of obstructing adenomatous tissue include the presence of a prominent, intravesical component, associated bladder pathology (ie, large, narrow-necked vesical diverticulum, multiple large bladder calculi), and the need for an open prostatectomy in an obese patient in whom the retropubic approach is technically more cumbersome.[5] Suprapubic prostatectomy is a relatively simple procedure that nevertheless requires meticulous attention to surgical detail.[6,7]

### Postoperative Hernia

A transverse (Pfannenstiel's) or lower midline incision may be used, depending upon the procedure planned, the patient's physique, and the presence of previous surgical scars. In the preferred Pfannenstiel's incision, avoid extending the incision too far laterally to decrease the risk of postoperative hernia.

### Missed Bladder Pathology or Injury

Careful examination of the opened bladder, especially to locate the trigone and the ureteral orifices and to identify associated bladder pathology, is important before enucleating the obstructing adenoma. A careful exploration at this juncture can prevent the need for re-exploration. The intraoperative use of intravenous (IV) chromagen dyes (eg, indocarmine, methylene blue) can ensure ureteral integrity.

### Injury to the Voluntary Sphincter

During the dissection portion of the procedure, the apex of the adenoma should be separated from the area adjacent to the external urethral sphincter bilaterally, leaving both lateral lobes free. The urethra then should be divided sharply or bluntly by pinching it proximal to the distal apical adenoma. Traction on the distal urethra should be avoided while the capsule is teased from the apex of the adenoma to minimize sphincter injury (see Figure 5-2).

### Intraoperative Bleeding

Post- and intraoperative bleeding remains a recurrent complication of open prostatectomy.[5] Introduction of a gauze pack into the prostatic fossa with blunt-tipped forceps, once a standard hemostatic procedure, is now used selectively as an excellent maneuver to achieve rapid control of significant bleeding. Place side-on (Halsted) hemostatic mattress sutures of absorbable suture incorporating bladder mucosa, bladder neck, and prostatic capsule at the 5 o'clock and 7 o'clock positions (Figure 7-1) is facilitated by use of a GU (five-eighths) curved needle. Persistent bleeding from deep in the posterior aspect of the

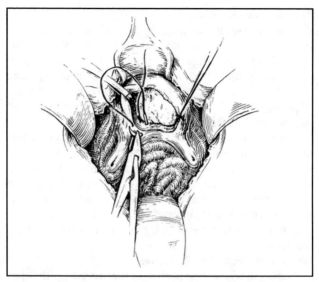

**Figure 7-1:** Hemostatic plication sutures. Persistent bleeding from the depths of the posterior prostatic fossa can be controlled by placing three transverse plication sutures of 0 chromic catgut. The sutures should engage the opposing lateral aspects of the fossa as well as the midzone component. Once tied, they induce an accordion-like effect, which facilitates hemostasis.

prostatic fossa can also be controlled by three transverse plication sutures of 0-chromic catgut placed in the prostatic fossa.[8] Before trigonalization of the prostatic fossa, a V-shaped wedge can be removed from the 6 o'clock area of the bladder neck, if it is extremely tight. Anchoring the bladder neck to the posterior aspect of the prostatic fossa facilitates hemostasis and prevents the formation of an obstructing membrane.

Problem bleeding has also been addressed by attempting direct visualization, suture or cautery control, and the use of hemostatic agents (ie, oxidized regenerated cellulose) placed in the prostatic fossa with temporary gauze packing or wrapped around the balloon. On rare occasions, an occlusive, preferably removable, pull-out suture of the bladder neck has been used.[9]

### Persistent Suprapubic Drainage

Persistent suprapubic drainage usually requires endoscopic and, at times, cystographic assessment to evaluate the possible presence of persistent obstructing tissue or a foreign body. Other, more remote causes may warrant consideration, if the fistula becomes chronic.

## Simple Open Retropubic Prostatectomy

Retropubic prostatectomy with a direct ventral capsulotomy can be used to permit a more exact adenomectomy and facilitate direct hemostasis.[10] Once the appropriate surgical plane has been entered, the enucleation of the obstructing adenoma is similar to that described for suprapubic prostatectomy. Larger glands are usually more easily enucleated with blunt-finger or closed scissor-tip dissection. The direct access to the prostatic fossa provided by the transcapsular incision facilitates the achievement of hemostasis. Similarly, retrigonalization of the bladder neck to the prostatic fossa should be considered to facilitate hemostasis, accelerate re-epithelization, prevent fibrosis, and aid future retrograde catheter manipulations.

Osteitis pubis is an uncommon postprostatectomy complication that can cause severe pain in the region of the symphysis, pelvis, or lower abdomen. Although most often associated with the retropubic approach, osteitis pubis can follow suprapubic and transurethral prostatectomy and even simple urethral instrumentation.[11] Symptoms usually begin within 6 weeks of the surgery. A low-grade fever, limited adduction of the thighs, and significant discomfort upon bilateral medially directed pelvic pressure raises suspicion of osteitis pubis. Radiographic changes in the bone, although not always present, are usually recognizable 2 to 4 weeks after the onset of symptoms.

## General Complications of Open Prostatectomy

Recent reports of short- and long-term experience with open prostatectomy are conspicuously lacking.[5] Consequently, improvements in morbidity and mortality that have occurred in the past two decades in surgical procedures in general are reflected minimally in the data available regarding open prostatectomy. The reports on open prostatectomy used for the 1994 Health Care Financing Administration (HCFA)/BPH guideline study summary[12] were published in 1987 or earlier. The mean perioperative mortality was 2.4% (90% confidence interval [CI] 1% to 4.6%), which compares with the progressively decreasing mortality rate from Northwestern University's Feinberg School of Medicine from 8.5% in 1942 to 1950, to 2.1% in 1961 to 1965, to 1.4% in 1965 to 1970, and finally 0% in 1971 to 1982.[5]

The mean and median overall complication rate (which is considered to be any complication regardless of severity) of open prostatectomy cited in the HCFA/BPH guideline is 21% (90% CI 7% to 42.7%). The 1.5% mean risk of perioperative intervention for bleeding and 35% mean risk of transfusion compares with 0.3% and 8%, respectively.[13] In the latter series, >50% of the patients undergoing transfusion received 1 unit of blood, an unlikely occurrence today. The guideline review indicated a mean incidence of 2.6% for epididymitis and 13.4% for UTI.

## Long-Term Complications

As reported in the HCFA/BPH guideline review of open prostatectomy, complications that usually lead to a prolonged follow-up include urethral stricture, with a mean incidence of 2.6%, and bladder neck contracture, with a mean incidence of 1.8%.[12] Both complications are reported to occur more frequently with a suprapubic than with a retropubic approach. The median risk of stress incontinence (retropubic 1.5%, suprapubic 2.6%) and total incontinence (retropubic 0.5%, suprapubic 0.3%) noted in the literature review seems to be relatively stable.

The HCFA/BPH guideline report[12] cites an estimated re-treatment rate of 2% (90% CI 1% to 4%) within 1 to 5 years following an open prostatectomy. No data are presented regarding the need for immediate intervention in patients who either are unable to void or have unimproved or worsened voiding dysfunction after surgical intervention.

Patients who are unable to void, have persistent drainage from the suprapubic site, unchanged or troublesome symptoms, or chronic UTI require prompt evaluation, usually including consideration of endoscopic, voiding cystourethrographic, and/or urodynamic studies. Although less common than after transurethral resection of the prostate (TURP), failure to remove obstructive BPH tissue may occur with open surgical procedures. Other factors, especially unsuspected neurogenic dysfunction, may be identified. In a HCFA-sponsored retrospective review of 2,617 Medicare patients undergoing a prostatectomy for BPH in 1985 (168 open, 2,449 TURP), the probability of reoperation in a 2-year period was 1.84% for patients undergoing open prostatectomy and 2.72% for those undergoing TURP.[14]

## Urinary Incontinence

Center studies report a low incidence of incontinence, ranging from 0% to 1.4% for both open and endoscopic procedures.[15,16] However, a prospective study by urologists in Maine of patients who had a prostatectomy reported that 4% had a problem with dripping or wet pants persisting for 1 year after the procedure.[17] This study also reported a 15% incidence of one or more episodes of AUR caused by blood clots within 3 months of surgery. The HCFA/BPH guideline review[12] indicates a median incidence of stress incontinence of 1.9% after open prostatectomy, 1.75% after transurethral incision of the prostate (TUIP), and 2.1% after TURP. The median incidence of total incontinence was 0.5%, 0.1%, and 1%, respectively.

## Sexual Dysfunction

Retrograde ejaculation is an anticipated phenomenon the incidence of which has been reported to vary from 30%

to 100%.[18,19] A mean probability of retrograde ejaculation of 24.9% for TUIP, 73.4% for TURP, and 77.2% for open prostatectomy reported in the HCFA/BPH guideline[12] supports the importance of a surgical approach and technique in the occurrence of this condition. In general, this postoperative sequela does not constitute a disabling problem for the elderly patient who is adequately prepared for its eventuality. In contrast to the incidence of postoperative retrograde ejaculation, most men who are sexually active and have a willing sexual partner preoperatively also maintain satisfactory erectile function after prostatic surgery. Finkle and Prian[20] reported potency rates of 95%, 87%, and 71% after transurethral, suprapubic, and perineal prostatectomies, respectively. Fowler et al[17] reported that 5% of the patients in their survey indicated a persistent inability to achieve erection after TURP. TUIP is associated with a 12% and TURP with a 14% incidence of postoperative erectile dysfunction (ED).

The varying indications for surgical intervention complicate the evaluation of BPH when rigid criteria are used, as does the knowledge that approximately 45% of patients treated with placebo and 40% treated with watchful waiting report overall symptomatic improvement.[12] The percentage of patients who judge their voiding symptoms as 'better' or 'much better' after surgery varies from 75% to 93%, depending on the severity of the patient's initial symptoms and the duration of follow-up treatment.[17,21,22] A review of the HCFA/BPH guideline[12] indicates an overall symptomatic improvement of 98% (90% CI 94% to 99.8%) for open prostatectomy, 88% (90% CI 75% to 96%) for TURP, and 80% (90% CI 78% to 83%) for TUIP. The guideline data review indicates that surgical procedures produced about an 80% improvement in symptom scores, appreciably higher than the 30% to 40% range for placebo and nonsurgical therapies. Nielsen[23] provides some evidence that the improved symptomatology is maintained in most patients for >7 years. In every series, some patient symptoms were unaffected by the prostatectomy, and some symptoms (3% to 12%) worsened. Although many practitioners have cautioned that patients with irritative, as opposed to obstructive, symptoms are at greater risk for poor results,[22] an evaluation by Jorgensen et al[24] failed to confirm this finding. Careful evaluation and selection are indicated in patients with predominantly irritative symptoms, and this may account for the good results (90%) from prostate surgery reported in the latter group of patients.

## References

1.    Foley SJ, Soloman LZ, Wedderburn AW, et al: A prospective study of the natural history of hematuria associated with benign prostatic hyperplasia and the effect of finasteride. *J Urol* 2000;163:496-498.

2.    Mebust WK, Holtgrewe HL, Cockett AT, et al: Transurethral prostatectomy: immediate and postoperative complications. A cooperative study of 13 participating institutions evaluating 3,885 patients. *J Urol* 2002;167:5-9.

3.    Hofer DR, Schaeffer AJ: Use of antimicrobials for patients undergoing prostatectomy. *Urol Clin North Am* 1990;17:595-600.

4.    Morris MJ, Golovsky D, Guinness MD, et al: The value of prophylactic antibiotics in transurethral prostatic resection: a controlled trial, with observations on the origin of postoperative infection. *Br J Urol* 1976;48:479-484.

5.    Helfand B, Mouli S, Dedhia R, et al: Management of lower urinary tract symptoms secondary to benign prostatic hyperplasia with open prostatectomy: results of a contemporary series. *J Urol* 2006;176(6 pt 1):2557-2561.

6.    Nanninga N, Brakenhoff GJ, Meijer M, et al: Bacterial anatomy in retrospect and prospect. *Antonie Van Leeuwenhoek* 1984;50:433-460.

7.    O'Conor VJ Jr: Review of experience with vesicovaginal fistula repair. *Trans Am Assoc Genitourin Surg* 1979;71:120-122.

8.    O'Conor VJ Jr: An aid for hemostasis in open prostatectomy: capsular plication. *J Urol* 1982;127:448.

9.    Malament M: Maximal hemostasis in suprapubic prostatectomy. *Surg Gynecol Obstet* 1965;120:1307-1312.

10.    Hodges CV, Barry JM: Suprapubic and retropubic prostatectomy for prostatic hyperlasia. *Urol Clin North Am* 1975;2:49-67.

163

11. Gangwal KC, Vickers P, Mathur SC: Osteitis pubis after prostatectomy. *Int Surg* 1971;56:18-22.

12. McConnell JD, Barry MJ, Bruskewitz RC: Benign prostatic hyperplasia: diagnosis and treatment. Agency for Health Care Policy and Research. *Clin Pract Guidel Quick Ref Guide Clin* 1994:1-17.

13. Nicoll GA, Riffle GN 2nd, Andersen FO: Suprapubic prostatectomy. The removable purse string: a continuing comparative analysis of 300 consecutive cases. *J Urol* 1978;120:702-704.

14. Taylor Z, Krakauer H: Mortality and reoperation following prostatectomy: outcomes in a Medicare population. *Urology* 1991;38 (suppl 1):27-31.

15. Holtgrewe HL, Valk WL: Late results of transurethral prostatectomy. *J Urol* 1964;92:51-55.

16. O'Conor VJ Jr, Bulkley GJ, Sokol JK: Low suprapubic prostatectomy: comparison of results with the standard operation in two comparable groups of 142 patients. *J Urol* 1963;90:301-304.

17. Fowler FJ Jr, Wennberg JE, Timothy RP, et al: Symptom status and quality of life following prostatectomy. *JAMA* 1988;259:3018-3022.

18. Caine M: The late results and sequelae of prostatectomy. *Br J Urol* 1954;26:205-226.

19. Melchior J, Valk WL, Foret JD, et al: Transurethral prostatectomy: computerized analysis of 2,223 consecutive cases. *J Urol* 1974;112:634-642.

20. Finkle AL, Prian DV: Sexual potency in elderly men before and after prostatectomy. *JAMA* 1966;196:139-143.

21. Bruskewitz RC, Larsen EH, Madsen PO, et al: 3-year follow-up of urinary symptoms after transurethral resection of the prostate. *J Urol* 1986;136:613-615.

22. Lepor H, Rigaud G: The efficacy of transurethral resection of the prostate in men with moderate symptoms of prostatism. *J Urol* 1990;143:533-537.

23. Nielsen KT, Christensen MM, Madsen PO, et al: Symptom analysis and uroflowmetry 7 years after transurethral resection of the prostate. *J Urol* 1989;142:1251-1253.

24. Jorgensen JB, Jensen KM, Mogensen P: Significance of predominantly irritative symptomatology before a prostatic operation. *J Urol* 1990;143:739-741.

# Chapter 8

# Complications of Minimally Invasive Treatments

ecause of its route of entry and potential injury to the urethra, prostate, and bladder, transurethral surgery (eg, interstitial laser coagulation [ILC], transurethral needle ablation [TUNA], transurethral resection of the prostate [TURP], visual laser ablation of the prostate [VLAP]) is predisposed to a unique set of possible complications not experienced with other forms of surgery. As such, vigilance is required to recognize and prevent these problems before they result in significant sequelae.

## Introduction of the Resectoscope/Instrumentation

To minimize intra- and postoperative complications, the resectoscope must be introduced into the bladder with minimal trauma to the urethra. However, certain pre- existing medical conditions may pose an obstacle. For example, phimosis may preclude entry of the resectoscope. In addition, the resectoscope may contribute to inadequate aseptic preparation of the glans itself, which may lead to severe urethritis, stricture formation, and possible postoperative sepsis secondary to trapped secretions. Cases such as these may warrant circumcision before surgical intervention for the treatment of benign prostatic hyperplasia (BPH).

Meatal stenosis is another pre-existing medical condition that could pose difficulties to resectoscope/instrument entrance. In addition, it may lead to severe urethral mucosal trauma if the instrument is forced into the bladder, resulting in postoperative meatal stricture formation,[1] which may be avoided with preoperative calibration of the urethra to define the degree of stenosis. A ventral meatotomy can be performed if sound dilation is not sufficient. Only in rare cases is internal urethrotomy or perineal urethrostomy required.

## Intraoperative Hemorrhage During Transurethral Surgery

It should be noted that patients undergoing surgical treatment for symptomatic BPH who have chosen an endourologic procedure (ie, TURP) would benefit from a preoperative course of 5α-reductase inhibitors (5ARIs), which has been shown to minimize bleeding during the procedure.[2] However, even with these medications, significant hemorrhage can occur in up to 20% of patients undergoing transurethral surgeries.[3]

Intraoperative bleeding can compromise visualization and therefore hinder tissue resection.[4] With a normal coagulation profile, the source of intraoperative bleeding is either open venous sinuses or an unidentified arterial source. The bladder neck usually constitutes the primary source of arterial bleeds because it houses the prostatic division of the inferior vesical arteries. When exposed, these pulsatile bleeding vessels must be immediately fulgurated.[5] It would also be prudent to re-examine this area at the termination of the procedure to prevent delayed identification of a postoperative hemorrhage site. The clinician should be cautious during fulguration to prevent damage to surrounding structures or perforation of bladder or urethral mucosa.

Intraoperative venous bleeding can generally be managed with cauterization.[6] Additionally, contraction of the prostatic capsule during resection aids in tamponade. In the setting of venous sinus bleeding, a different course of action must be undertaken because further cauterization may only exacerbate the vessel defect and intensify the degree of bleeding. To avoid such instances, the clinician should take care to resect prostatic tissue in smooth planes, avoiding deep bites that can result in such complications.[5] If a venous sinus begins to hemorrhage during the procedure, do not increase the rate of fluid irrigation. This will only increase absorption of irrigating fluid and theoretically increase the risk of transurethral resection (TUR) syndrome (see below). Instead, the resectoscope should be used to tamponade the bleeding site, thereby improving visualization. Placing a urethral catheter balloon on tension also can provide additional hemostasis.

## Trauma to Landmarks

Many transurethral technologies resect prostatic adenoma and subsequently relieve a patient's bladder outlet obstruction (BOO) and lower urinary tract symptoms (LUTS). However, even under direct visualization, other nonprostatic tissue may be at risk for resection or injury.[7] For example, in the setting of trigonal hypertrophy, the ureteral orifices are displaced toward the prostate, putting them at risk during prostatic resection or the processes of prostatic energy application. The prostate adenomatous tissue itself may also obscure the orifices, as can advanced trabeculation with diverticula. If ureteral resection or fulguration of the ureteral orifices occurs, patients must be monitored for subsequent obstruction, hydronephrosis, and/or stricture formation. To avoid such trauma, visualizing the orifices before resecting, as well as intermittently during the procedure, is recommended. Indigo carmine may be used to identify the orifices if they are not readily seen with the resectoscope or camera. Indigo carmine should also be used to identify the ureteral orifices at the end of resecting if they are not clearly visible.

To avoid inadvertent trauma to the external sphincter, the clinician should maintain visualization of the verumontanum.[6] The apex of the prostate lies adjacent to the verumontanum, and residual tissue here may cause postoperative voiding dysfunction. The anterior-most portion of the adenomatous tissue can be found at the level of the verumontanum. Resection can often be extended too far distally at this location, and care must be taken to avoid this potential pitfall.

## Urethral Perforation During Transurethral Surgery

Perforation of the urethra or the prostate, which can occur at any time during the course of tissue resection or energy application, can be caused by unintentional manipulation of the instruments used for minimally invasive treatments (MITs).[8,9] The risk of perforation is further increased with established urethral strictures or false passages. To avoid this complication, the resectoscope or instrument should be passed under direct vision and placement of the device confirmed. Perforation or injury to the distal urethra may be managed conservatively by Foley catheter placement.

Deep-tissue resection at the level of the bladder neck can also cause perforation because this area is not protected by a large amount of adenomatous tissue. Therefore, injury to the urethra and bladder has been reported in many transurethral surgeries used to treat BPH.[10,11] To avoid such damage, it is recommended that resection be performed with a partially filled bladder and that particular care be taken to limit resection to adenomatous tissue.

Lateral and anterior perforation of the bladder and/or bladder neck can result in significant extravasation of irrigating fluid.[11] It is often difficult to visualize perforations at these sites, but absence of fluid return and diminished maneuverability of the resectoscope should raise suspicions of these complications. Other signs of perforation include elevation and compression of the lateral borders of the bladder with poor visualization of the bladder neck. In addition, patients with extraperitoneal extravasation of fluid may experience TUR syndrome (see below) with nausea, vomiting, abdominal pain, mental status changes, hypotension, tachycardia, diaphoresis, and dyspnea. Physical signs include abdominal rigidity and tenderness. With the advent of TUR syndrome, the procedure should be terminated (ie, after hemostasis is achieved, and resected tissue has been removed), and a urethral catheter inserted. Suprapubic drainage of the retroperitoneum may be warranted to minimize further fluid absorption.

Intraperitoneal extravasation can occur with bladder perforation during transurethral surgery. This will cause an abnormal irrigating pattern, with more irrigating fluid entering the bladder than is recovered. Symptoms are similar to the aforementioned extraperitoneal extravasation but are much more prominent. In such cases, laparotomy and peritoneal drainage should be limited to patients exhibiting respiratory compromise, or to cases of suspected bowel trauma. Less acute scenarios may be managed with catheter drainage and diuretics.

## TUR Syndrome

Historically, TUR syndrome has been reported in from 1% to 7% of patients undergoing TURP.[12] However, many of the newer MITs and newer biopolar TURP techniques do not have the same frequency. Despite this fact, excessive absorption of irrigating fluid during any transurethral surgery could theoretically result in TUR syndrome.[13] Therefore, it is important to recognize the constellation of features associated with this syndrome, including hypertension, bradycardia, restlessness, muscle twitching, disorientation, visual disturbances, seizures, and vascular collapse.[8,14,15]

Early recognition of TUR syndrome permits early management and may prevent the full spectrum of the syndrome.[14] Initial treatment may include a small suprapubic incision with insertion of a Penrose drain to permit fluid drainage. To mobilize fluid that has already been absorbed, hypertonic saline may be administered (200 to 500 mL of 1.8% to 5% solution) with intravenous (IV) furosemide (40 to 100 mg). Central venous pressure and urine output must be carefully and regularly monitored with the addition of hypertonic saline because this substance adds volume to an already taxed circulatory system. Serum electrolytes and osmolarity should also be monitored closely. Patients with end-stage renal disease (ESRD) may present with symptomatic hyponatremia even in the absence of serum hypo-osmolality. In these cases, dialysis may be warranted to elevate serum sodium and reduce the osmolar gap produced by absorbed sorbitol.

Replacement with 5% dextrose/0.5% normal saline can also be used to manage TUR syndrome.[14] If urine output is <250 mL/hour, the entire amount of fluid loss should be replaced. If urine outputs range from 250 to 500 mL/hour, then fluid replacement should be two thirds of this volume. Outputs >500 mL/hour should be replaced with 50% of the hourly volume. Total fluid replacement should not be 1,500 to 2,000 mL less than the total urine output. Frequent measurement of both serum and urine electrolytes is necessary.

## Perioperative and Postoperative Complications

### Perioperative Fever

Fever following transurethral surgery for the treatment of BPH may suggest bacteremia. Preoperative antibiotics may prevent this scenario and should be routinely used for transurethral surgery. In particular, antibiotics should be given preoperatively to patients with existing urinary tract infections (UTIs), prior indwelling catheterization, and prior instrumentation. If these measures are taken preoperatively, a change in antibiotics following the development of a postoperative fever is not indicated.[16,17] If prophylactic preoperative antibiotics have not been used, bacteriuria can be prevented by undertaking several measures. For example, a closed drainage system should be used, but frequent catheterization and continuous bladder irrigation should be avoided.

Nonsterile technique, phimosis, and bacterial contamination of instruments may also contribute to perioperative cystitis, which is amenable to antibiotic treatment. Prophylactic antibiotics may decrease the risk of postoperative cystitis. In diabetic patients, cystitis may be secondary to yeast colonization in the presence of indwelling catheterization and antibiotic treatment. These patients require administration of antifungal medications, including amphotericin B (Abelcet®, Ambisome®, Amphotec®, Fungizone®) or 5-fluocytosine to eradicate the infection. To circumvent this complication in at-risk patients, early removal of indwelling catheters is necessary.

Acute prostatitis and pyelonephritis are rare in the perioperative period. Acute epididymitis, however, may be observed especially if an indwelling catheter has been in place for an extended period.[16] In fact, epididymitis is also particularly common in patients who undergo instrumentation while they are bacteriuric. Most cases of epididymitis after urologic surgery are caused by gram-negative bacilli (eg, *Escherichia coli*, *Pseudomonas aeruginosa*, *Klebsiella*, *Enterobacter*). Extended treatment with antibiotics is recommended in this scenario.

Urethritis frequently occurs at a rate of about 1% following MITs for BOO due to BPH. Perioperative staphylococcal urethritis may occur between 4 and 5 days postoperatively, most often secondary to use of an indwelling catheter. Treatment may be instituted by removal of the indwelling catheter and the use of antibiotics (ie, penicillin or cephalexin [Keflex®]).

### Shock

Hypovolemic shock may develop in the setting of bacteremia and sepsis.[17,18] The most common cause of septic shock in this setting is prior infection with *E coli*, *Klebsiella*, *Bacteroides*, or *Pseudomonas*, any of which can gain access to the bloodstream during resection or in the postoperative period.

Patients will present with fever, rigors, and altered mental status. Additional signs include hypotension, oliguria, decreased central venous pressure, decreased cardiac output, tachycardia, metabolic acidosis, respiratory alkalosis, and occasional disseminated intravascular coagulation. Septic shock in the elderly may present more subtly, exhibiting fever only after electrolyte and fluid disturbances are severe enough to produce cardiogenic shock. Further complications include respiratory distress syndrome, acute renal failure, and heart failure.

### Irritative Symptoms

Following many of the MITs mentioned above, patients may experience urinary frequency, urinary urgency, dysuria, occasional urge incontinence, and weak urinary stream.[19,20] Depending on the type of MIT employed, these symptoms are often limited in duration and abate 6 to 8 weeks postoperatively. Therefore, patients presenting with these postoperative complaints usually require only reassurance. However, in certain circumstances, irritative voiding symptoms should mandate closer attention. For example, if irritative symptoms persist for >6 months postoperatively, evaluation for a neoplasm of the bladder or upper urinary tract must be undertaken. Persistent hematuria also requires similar investigation. If further evaluation is unremarkable (ie, revealing only inflammatory changes in the remaining prostatic tissue or trigone), patients may be amenable to conservative therapy (ie, antispasmodics).

Depending on the type of surgery performed, irritative voiding symptoms may also be a sign of inadequate resection. Therefore, cystoscopic evaluation should be undertaken if a patient continues to have persistent irritative voiding symptoms and/or LUTS postoperatively.

### Incontinence

Incontinence following transurethral surgery has multiple etiologies, including inflammation, neoplasm, residual tissue, or intrinsic weakness of the external urethral sphincter or detrusor instability. Evaluation in any of these circumstances includes urinalysis, urine culture, cystourethroscopy, and urodynamic studies.

The most common type of incontinence presenting after prostatic resection is urge incontinence. It is believed that this type of incontinence occurs secondary to inflammatory changes and/or may be related to the prostatic fossa. Stress incontinence may occur if the external sphincter or tissue adjacent to the verumontanum has been damaged. Furthermore, damage to the external sphincter may result in scarring with subsequent urethral stricture formation. If such stricture formation prevents complete closure of the sphincter mechanism, incontinence will result. This may be prevented with urethral sound dilation; however, the physician must take care to avoid undermining the bladder neck and creating false passages. If necessary, direct-vision urethrotomy may be used. In the setting of minor stress incontinence, patients may be amenable to undertaking an exercise regimen to enhance the voluntary closure of the external sphincter.

Patients who are not amenable to these measures may require some form of catheterization. Indwelling catheterization may be preferable in the elderly, who may not tolerate external collection devices. In some instances, a suprapubic catheter may be the best option. Additionally, several surgical options have been developed to treat urinary incontinence.

### Strictures/Contractures Following MITs

As mentioned above, transurethral surgeries and MITs induce inflammation and injury to the urethra, prostate, and surrounding structures. This inflammation can lead to scar and/or stricture formation. Bladder neck contractures are one type of stricture occurring secondary to the resection of the bladder neck.[21] The management of bladder neck contractures is determined by the degree of contracture. Most contractures may be managed by transurethral inci-

***Treatment***

Circumcision

Sound dilation or ventral meatotomy

Fulguration/supportive care/close monitoring of vitals/ blood transfusion

Verify with indigo carmine/possible stent/possible reconstruction/possible reimplantation depending on location and degree of trauma

1. Distal urethra→Foley catheter placement

2. Proximal urethra/bladder neck→Determine if intra- or extraperitoneal extravasation (obtain cystogram if necessary)

   a. Extraperitoneal, then Foley placement

   b. Intraperitoneal, then open exploration and repair

Close monitoring with vital signs and laboratory tests, hypertonic saline/sodium replacement

*continued on next page*

8

sion. However, in cases of severe disease, an open Y-V plasty may be necessary to alleviate symptoms.

Urethral strictures can also occur following transurethral surgery.[22-24] The most common locations of these scar formations are at the level of the membranous urethra, bulbar urethra at the penoscrotal junction, and fossa navicularis.

**Table 8-1: Quick Reference to Common Complications and Treatments Related to Minimally Invasive Treatments for Symptomatic BPH** (continued)

Peri- and Postoperative

*Complication*

UTI/bacteremia/sepsis

Irritative voiding symptoms

Hematuria

Incontinence

Urethral strictures

UTI=urinary tract infection

Patients with urethral strictures usually present with progressive obstructive symptoms. Depending on the severity of outflow obstruction, such symptoms can be managed with either urethral dilation or internal urethrotomy under direct visualization. Only rarely will open urethroplasty be necessary.

As mentioned above, stricture formation can be minimized by preventing urethral trauma during surgery. Postoperative catheter selection can also minimize the formation of strictures. Silastic catheters are less traumatic to the urethral mucosa and may be beneficial in select cases. Additionally,

### Treatment

Culture and treat with antibiotics, supportive care.

May be benign or managed supportively in perioperative period. However, if it persists, then should evaluate cystoscopically.

May be benign or managed supportively in perioperative period. However, if it persists, evaluate by cystoscopy and radiograph.

Evaluate for UTI, and, if needed, by cystourethroscopy and urodynamics.

Management should be determined by degree of stricture and may include dilation, incision, or open Y-V plasty.

when placed, the catheter should not place tension on either the bladder neck or the urethra at the penoscrotal junction to minimize contracture and stricture formation.

## Conclusions

MITs are promising alternatives to the more traditional open surgical treatments for BPH. However, they are not without morbidities (Table 8-1). It is important to screen for complications and have an understanding of the management of the complications following transurethral MITs for symptomatic BPH. Furthermore, physicians must consider the frequency of these complications and the potential for retreatment when choosing a MIT instead of an open surgical treatment.

## References

1.    Fourcade RO, Vallancien G: [Morbidity of endoscopic prostatic resection: 3-month prospective study. Practical Urology Club]. *Prog Urol* 2000;10:48-52.

2.    Ozdal OL, Ozden C, Benli K, et al: Effect of short-term finasteride therapy on peroperative bleeding in patients who were candidates for transurethral resection of the prostate (TUR-P): a randomized controlled study. *Prostate Cancer Prostatic Dis* 2005;8:215-218.

3.    Mebust WK, Holtgrewe HL, Cockett AT, et al: Transurethral prostatectomy: immediate and postoperative complications. A cooperative study of 13 participating institutions evaluating 3,885 patients. *J Urol* 1989;141:243-247.

4.    Grayhack JT, McVary KT, Kozlowski JM: *Benign Prostatic Hyperplasia*. Philadelphia, PA, Lippincott Williams & Wilkins, 2002, pp 1401-1470.

5.    Berger AP, Wirtenberger W, Bektic J, et al: Safer transurethral resection of the prostate: coagulating intermittent cutting reduces hemostatic complications. *J Urol* 2004;171:289-291.

6.    May F, Hartung R: Surgical atlas. Transurethral resection of the prostate. *BJU Int* 2006;98:921-934.

7.    Martov AG, Kornienko SI, Gushchin BL, et al: [Intraoperative urological complications in transurethral surgical interventions on the prostate for benign hyperplasia]. *Urologiia* 2005;4:3-8.

8.    AUA guideline on the management of benign prostatic hyperplasia (2003). Chapter 1: Diagnosis and treatment recommendations. *J Urol* 2003;170(2 pt 1):530-547.

9.    Uchida T, Adachi K, Ao T, et al: [Pre-operative, operative and postoperative complications in 2266 cases of transurethral resection of the prostate]. *Nippon Hinyokika Gakkai Zasshi* 1993;84: 897-905.

10.   Kuo RL, Kim SC, Lingeman JE, et al: Holmium laser enucleation of prostate (HoLEP): the Methodist Hospital experience with greater than 75 gram enucleations. *J Urol* 2003;170:149-152.

11.   Kolozsy Z, Csapo Z: [Bladder neck perforations caused by TURP (transurethral prostatectomy)]. *Z Urol Nephrol* 1983;76:65-73.

12. Hahn RG: Transurethral resection syndrome from extravascular absorption of irrigating fluid. *Scand J Urol Nephrol* 1993;27: 387-394.

13. Hahn RG: Fluid absorption in endoscopic surgery. *Br J Anaesth* 2006;96:8-20.

14. Berges RR, Pientka L: Management of the BPH syndrome in Germany: who is treated and how? *Eur Urol* 1999;36(suppl 3): 21-27.

15. Hahn RG: The transurethral resection syndrome. *Acta Anaesthesiol Scand* 1991;35:557-567.

16. Smith RB, Erhrlich RM: *Complications of Urologic Surgery: Prevention and Management*, 2nd ed. Philadelphia, PA, WB Saunders Co, 1990.

17. Qiang W, Jianchen W, MacDonald R, et al: Antibiotic prophylaxis for transurethral prostatic resection in men with preoperative urine containing less than 100,000 bacteria per ml: a systematic review. *J Urol* 2005;173:1175-1181.

18. Smith MS, Schambra UB, Wilson KH, et al: Alpha1-adrenergic receptors in human spinal cord: specific localized expression of mRNA encoding alpha1-adrenergic receptor subtypes at four distinct levels. *Brain Res Mol Brain Res* 1999;63:254-261.

19. Rubeinstein JN, McVary KT: Transurethral microwave thermotherapy for benign prostatic hyperplasia. *Int Braz J Urol* 2003;29: 251-263.

20. Wasson JH, Bubolz TA, Lu-Yao GL, et al: Transurethral resection of the prostate among medicare beneficiaries: 1984 to 1997. For the Patient Outcomes Research Team for Prostatic Diseases. *J Urol* 2000;164:1212-1215.

21. Lee YH, Chiu AW, Huang JK: Comprehensive study of bladder neck contracture after transurethral resection of prostate. *Urology* 2005;65:498-503; discussion 503.

22. Stormont TJ, Suman VJ, Oesterling JE: Newly diagnosed bulbar urethral strictures: etiology and outcome of various treatments. *J Urol* 1993;150(5 pt 2):1725-1728.

23. Nielsen KK, Nordling J: Urethral stricture following transurethral prostatectomy. *Urology* 1990;35:18-24.

24. Lentz HC Jr, Mebust WK, Foret JD, et al: Urethral strictures following transurethral prostatectomy: review of 2,223 resections. *J Urol* 1977;117:194-196.

# Chapter 9

# Phytotherapy

P hytotherapy is the use of plants or plant extracts for medical therapy. Plant extracts have been used for treating symptoms related to benign prostatic hyperplasia (BPH) since ancient times. The use and prevalence of phytotherapy for symptomatic BPH are influenced by geographic location. Although not as prevalent in the United States, phytotherapy is widely used in Europe. For example, in Germany, up to 90% of all patients with BPH are treated with phytopharmaceutical agents, and it has been reported that about half of all German urologists prefer plant-based therapies over chemically derived therapies.[1]

Although these phytotherapeutic agents have been used in Europe for centuries, little is known about the true mechanism of action that gives them therapeutic abilities. Several factors have affected their acceptance for use in the treatment of lower urinary tract symptoms (LUTS) due to BPH.[2] For example, only a limited number of randomized, double-blind trials have been conducted using phytotherapies; therefore, most studies have been uncontrolled, and the possibility of a placebo effect cannot be ruled out. In addition, the active ingredient in most of these plant extracts is unknown because of the abundance of compounds contained in them, making direct comparison between medications nearly impossible. Finally, most previously reported studies did not use standardized urinary symptom scores (ie, the American Urological Association-

International Prostate Symptom Score [AUA-IPSS]) in their evaluation of efficacy, which also makes quantitation and direct comparison difficult.

Despite these problems, many phytotherapies are available and marketed for the treatment of BPH. In fact, approximately 30 different phytotherapeutic compounds are used for the treatment of BPH; some of the major ones are examined below and are listed in Table 9-1.

## Saw Palmetto (Serenoa repens)

Extract from the saw palmetto (*Serenoa repens*) plant is the most widely used phytotherapeutic agent for BPH. Saw palmetto is a dwarf palm tree native to the West Indies and the southeastern United States. It was initially used by Native Americans to increase testicular function and relieve genitourinary irritation.[2] The lipid-soluble components of saw palmetto berries are believed to contain the active components for the treatment of BPH.[2] The purified lipid extract is used medicinally and consists of fatty acids and sterols, such as β-sitosterol. However, the exact mechanism by which these compounds exert their anti-androgen effects and relieve LUTS remains to be determined.

Throughout the past two decades, substantial literature has emerged examining the biologic and clinical effects of saw palmetto extracts.[3-5] Some clinical studies have attempted to compare the effects of saw palmetto with the 5α-reductase inhibitor (5ARI) finasteride (Proscar®), as well as with the α-adrenergic receptor antagonists alfuzosin (Uroxatral®) and tamsulosin (Flomax®).[6,7] Results from these studies have suggested that saw palmetto may have some efficacy in increasing peak urinary flow rate ($Q_{max}$).

However, many of the published studies demonstrate inconclusive results because of problems with inclusion/exclusion criteria, lack of a uniform symptom score analysis, lack of power, lack of a placebo run-in period, and short duration of therapy. When the appropriate controls have

## Table 9-1: Available Phytotherapeutic Agents Used for the Treatment of BPH

| Plant | Common Name | Trade Name |
|-------|-------------|------------|
| *Serenoa repens* | Saw palmetto | Permixon |
| *Pygeum africanum* | African plum | Tadenan |
| *Secale cereale* | Rye-grass pollen | Cernilton |
| *Hypoxis rooperi* | South African star grass | Harzol |
| *Pinus picea* | Pine flower spruce | Azurusat (combination) |

There are many compounds contained within plant extracts; thus, the true chemical nature of these extracts is generally unclear. The *active agent* designation in this table is only proposed. In general, the components of plant extracts are phytosterols, phytoestrogens, and terpenoids.[8,9] Unfortunately, many of the reported studies

been used, the clinical value of saw palmetto for treating LUTS has come into question.[10-13] For example, a recent double-blind trial randomized 225 men with moderate-to-severe symptoms of BPH to 1 year of treatment with saw palmetto extract (160 mg twice a day) or placebo.[12] The primary outcome measures were changes in the scores on the American Urological Association Symptom Index (AUA-SI) and in $Q_{max}$. Secondary outcome measures included changes in prostate size, postvoid residual urine (PVR) volume, quality of life (QOL), laboratory values,

| Proposed Active Agent | Proposed Method of Action |
|---|---|
| Fatty acids, sterols | Anti-androgen Anti-β-FGF, Anti-EGF |
| β-sitosterol | Cholesterol mechanism |
| Fatty alcohols | Inhibits β-FGF |
| Fatty acids | EGH |
| | Anti-inflammatory |
| β-sterols | Anti-androgen |
| | Inhibitors of prostaglandins |
| | Leukotriene synthesis |
| β-sitosterol | Anti-inflammatory |
| | Anticholesterol metabolism |
| β-sitosterol | Anti-inflammatory |
| | Anticholesterol metabolism |

that have evaluated the mechanisms of action of plant extracts have used supraphysiologic doses.[8,9] In addition, many of these studies have failed to be double blind and placebo controlled.

β-FGF=β-fibroblast growth factor; EGF=epidermal growth factor; EGH=equine growth hormone; FGF=fibroblast growth factor

and the rate of reported adverse effects. When these parameters were evaluated after 1 year, there was no significant difference between the saw palmetto and placebo groups in the change in AUA-SI scores, $Q_{max}$, prostate size, PVR volume, QOL, or serum prostate-specific antigen (PSA) levels (Table 9-2).

Clinical studies have shown a low frequency of side effects attributed to the use of saw palmetto for the treatment of symptomatic BPH. Adverse effects associated with saw palmetto are generally mild and comparable with placebo.

## Table 9-2: Outcomes of Saw Palmetto for the Treatment of BPH

| Measure | Saw Palmetto (N=112) |
|---|---|
| American Urological Association Symptom Index (AUA-SI) | -0.68 ± 0.35 |
| Peak urinary flow rate ($Q_{max}$) (mL/sec) | 0.42 ± 0.34 |
| Postvoid residual urine (PVR) volume (mL) | 14.10 ± 7.24 |
| Sexual function (O'Leary scale) | -0.06 ± 0.10 |

One of the first, large, double-blind trials evaluating saw palmetto for the treatment of BPH demonstrated no significant difference in outcomes between saw palmetto and placebo.[12]

Generally, *Serenoa repens* has a slightly lower rate of side effects compared with more traditional therapies[14] (Table 9-3). Acute urinary retention (AUR) occurred at the same rate in both the saw palmetto and tamsulosin groups.

### African Plum Tree Extract (*Pygeum africanum*)

*Pygeum africanum*, another phytotherapy, is derived from the African plum tree,[4] and has been used in Europe for more than 50 years to treat genitourinary symptoms. Like many of the other phytotherapies, the mechanism of action of *P africanum* is not known. However, researchers have postulated that the active components in the extract include phytosterols, especially β-sitosterols, and long chain fatty alcohols. In animal studies, these compounds are believed to modulate bladder contractility, decrease inflammation, and decrease the production of leukotrienes.[15]

Figure 9-1 represents data obtained from one randomized, placebo-controlled trial, involving 263 patients, which

| Placebo (N=113) | Difference Between Groups (95% confidence interval [CI]) |
|---|---|
| -0.7 2 ± 0.35 | 0.04 |
| -0.01 ± 0.34 | 0.43 |
| 18.62 ± 7.14 | -4.51 |
| 0.07 ± 0.10 | -0.13 |

evaluated the efficacy of African plum tree extract. The data suggest that African plum tree extract can improve urinary symptoms when compared with placebo.[16] Results from a meta-analysis of clinical studies of *P africanum* indicate that it modestly improves urologic symptoms and urinary flow (uroflow) rates.[17] However, like the other phytotherapies, further research involving multicenter, randomized, placebo-controlled studies are needed to determine its long-term effectiveness and efficacy in the treatment of LUTS due to BPH.

## Rye-grass Pollen (Secale cereale)

Rye-grass pollen extract (Cernilton) is another phytotherapy that has been applied to the treatment of symptomatic BPH. In the United States, rye-grass pollen extract is used by approximately 5,000 men daily.[18] One dose of Cernilton contains 60 mg of water-soluble compounds and approximately 3 mg of acetone-soluble compounds.

## Table 9-3: Adverse Effects of Phytotherapy: A Comparison Between Saw Palmetto and Tamsulosin[14]

| Adverse Effect | Saw Palmetto (%) | Tamsulosin (%) |
|---|---|---|
| Rhinitis | 8.6 | 12.1 |
| Headache | 8.0 | 10.5 |
| Dizziness | 2.9 | 1.7 |
| Fatigue | 1.7 | 1.4 |
| Asthenia | 1.1 | 1.4 |
| Hypotension (postural) | 1.1 | <1.0 |
| Dry mouth | <1.0 | <1.0 |
| Ejaculatory disorders | <1.0 | 4.2 |
| Decrease in libido | <1.0 | 1.1 |

The rate of adverse reactions to saw palmetto is low and comparable to the $\alpha$-adrenergic antagonist tamsulosin.

The acetone-soluble fraction contains $\beta$-sterols, which are believed to be the active components of the extract responsible for the anti-androgen and muscle-relaxing properties of rye-grass pollen extract.

A systematic review of the literature indicates that rye-grass pollen extract can decrease the frequency of nocturia and reduce the PVR volume in patients with BPH. Rye-grass pollen extract had no more effect than placebo or active controls on uroflow measures.[19] Overall, it remains to be determined whether rye-grass pollen extract is efficacious in the treatment of BPH. Randomized, placebo-controlled, multicenter studies are required to determine rye-grass pollen extract's effectiveness.

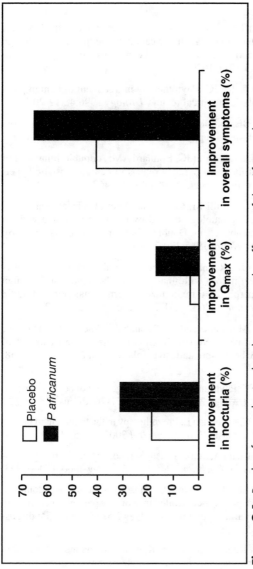

**Figure 9-1:** Results of a randomized trial comparing the efficacy of the African plum tree extract *Pygeum africanum* with placebo for the treatment of patients with BPH.[16] The data obtained from this relatively small trial suggest that *P africanum* extract has some efficacy in treating LUTS due to BPH. BPH=benign prostatic hyperplasia; LUTS=lower urinary tract symptoms; $Q_{max}$ =peak urinary flow rate

# References

1.    Krzeski T, Kazon M, Borkowski A, et al: Combined extracts of Urtica dioica and Pygeum africanum in the treatment of benign prostatic hyperplasia: double-blind comparison of two doses. *Clin Ther* 1993;15:1011-1020.

2.    Lowe FC, Ku JC: Phytotherapy in treatment of benign prostatic hyperplasia: a critical review. *Urology* 1996;48:12-20.

3.    Carbin BE, Larsson B, Lindahl O: Treatment of benign prostatic hyperplasia with phytosterols. *Br J Urol* 1990;66:639-641.

4.    Champault G, Patel JC, Bonnard AM: A double-blind trial of an extract of the plant Serenoa repens in benign prostatic hyperplasia. *Br J Clin Pharmacol* 1984;18:461-462.

5.    Tasca A, Barulli M, Cavazzana A, et al: [Treatment of obstructive symptomatology caused by prostatic adenoma with an extract of Serenoa repens. Double-blind clinical study vs. placebo]. *Minerva Urol Nefrol* 1985;37:87-91.

6.    Carraro JC, Raynaud JP, Koch G, et al: Comparison of phytotherapy (Permixon) with finasteride in the treatment of benign prostate hyperplasia: a randomized international study of 1,098 patients. *Prostate* 1996;29:231-240; discussion 241-242.

7.    Grasso M, Montesano A, Buonaguidi A, et al: Comparative effects of alfuzosin versus Serenoa repens in the treatment of symptomatic benign prostatic hyperplasia. *Arch Esp Urol* 1995;48: 97-103.

8.    Lowe FC: Phytotherapy in the management of benign prostatic hyperplasia. *Urology* 2001;58(suppl 1):71-76; discussion 76-77.

9.    Lowe FC, Fagelman E: Phytotherapy in the treatment of benign prostatic hyperplasia. *Curr Opin Urol* 2002;12:15-18.

10.    Wilt T, Ishani A, Stark G, et al: Serenoa repens for benign prostatic hyperplasia. *Cochrane Database Syst Rev* 2000; CD001423.

11.    Gerber GS, Kuznetsov D, Johnson BC, et al: Randomized, double-blind, placebo-controlled trial of saw palmetto in men with lower urinary tract symptoms. *Urology* 2001;58:960-964; discussion 964-965.

12.    Bent S, Kane C, Shinohara K, et al: Saw palmetto for benign prostatic hyperplasia. *N Engl J Med* 2006;354:557-566.

13. Willetts KE, Clements MS, Champion S, et al: Serenoa repens extract for benign prostate hyperplasia: a randomized controlled trial. *BJU Int* 2003;92:267-270.

14. Boyle P, Robertson C, Lowe F, et al: Updated meta-analysis of clinical trials of Serenoa repens extract in the treatment of symptomatic benign prostatic hyperplasia. *BJU Int* 2004;93:751-756.

15. Wilt T, Ishani A, MacDonald R, et al: Pygeum africanum for benign prostatic hyperplasia. *Cochrane Database Syst Rev* 2002; CD001044.

16. Barlet A, Albrecht J, Aubert A, et al: [Efficacy of Pygeum africanum extract in the medical therapy of urination disorders due to benign prostatic hyperplasia: evaluation of objective and subjective parameters. A placebo-controlled double-blind multicenter study]. *Wien Klin Wochenschr* 1990;102:667-673.

17. Ishani A, MacDonald R, Nelson D, et al: Pygeum africanum for the treatment of patients with benign prostatic hyperplasia: a systematic review and quantitative meta-analysis. *Am J Med* 2000; 109:654-664.

18. Wilt TJ, Ishani A, Rutks I, et al: Phytotherapy for benign prostatic hyperplasia. *Public Health Nutr* 2000;3:459-472.

19. MacDonald R, Ishani A, Rutks I, et al: A systematic review of Cernilton for the treatment of benign prostatic hyperplasia. *BJU Int* 2000;85:836-841.

9

# Chapter 10

# Investigational Therapies for BPH

The main goal of treatment for benign prostatic hyperplasia (BPH) is relief of bothersome voiding symptoms. Medical therapy with antiadrenergic or antiandrogenic medications is often the initial treatment, and transurethral resection of the prostate (TURP) continues to be the most common surgical procedure. Minimally invasive treatments (MITs) offer an alternative for patients who do not wish to remain on medication or who are not suitable candidates for surgery.

Medical therapy for BPH approved by the US Food and Drug Administration (FDA) includes $\alpha$-adrenergic receptor blockers such as alfuzosin (Uroxatral®), doxazosin (Cardura®, Cardura® XL), tamsulosin (Flomax®), and terazosin (Hytrin®), and 5$\alpha$-reductase inhibitors (5ARIs) finasteride (Proscar®) and dutasteride (Avodart®). Both classes of drugs are effective in reducing symptom severity and bother, but each has side effects that occasionally cause patients to discontinue therapy (Table 10-1). The side effects of $\alpha$-blocker therapy may include hypotension, dizziness, orthostasis, fatigue, somnolence, and retrograde ejaculation.[1,2] Sexual side effects such as erectile dysfunction (ED), decreased libido, and decreased ejaculatory volume[3,4] are more commonly associated with the 5ARIs. The goal of investigational therapeutic options is increased efficacy with fewer and less bothersome side effects. This

## Table 10-1: Side Effects of α-Blockers and 5ARIs

| α-Blockers | 5ARIs |
|---|---|
| • hypotension | • ED |
| • dizziness | • ejaculatory dysfunction |
| • orthostasis | • decreased libido |
| • fatigue | |
| • somnolence | |
| • retrograde ejaculation | |
| • erectile dysfunction (ED) | |
| • headache | |
| • asthenia | |
| • rhinitis | |

5ARIs=5α-reductase inhibitors

chapter examines some of the investigational treatments for BPH not yet approved by the FDA.

## Phosphodiesterase Inhibitors

Phosphodiesterase (PDE) inhibitors, and specifically inhibitors of the PDE-5 isoenzyme, are approved by the FDA for the treatment of ED in men. Now the PDE-5 inhibitors are among the medical therapies under study for treatment of lower urinary tract symptoms (LUTS) due to BPH. The prostate gland enlarges with advancing age, as does the prevalence of LUTS and ED.[5,6] Patients with LUTS frequently also have ED and those with ED frequently experience LUTS. The PDE-5-inhibiting drugs sildenafil (Viagra®), vardenafil (Levitra®), and tadalafil (Cialis®) relax the smooth muscle of the corpus cavernosum tissue of the penis, which is an essential step in the process of erection.

The mechanism of action begins when nerve terminals release the neurotransmitter nitric oxide (NO). NO stimulates synthesis of cyclic guanosine monophosphate (cGMP), which initiates dilation of the cavernosus smooth muscle.[7] Inhibitors of the PDE enzymes, as well as NO donors, are agents that elevate intracellular levels of cGMP and, therefore, enhance the erectile process.

PDE-5 is also abundant in the prostate, where it may regulate smooth muscle tone through much the same mechanism of action as in the cavernosal tissue. The drugs that are used to treat ED are now being studied for the treatment of LUTS and BPH. Results are promising from preliminary studies that sought to determine if PDE-5 acts on the prostate to reduce prostatic smooth muscle tone. Takeda and colleagues[8] led the way in research on PDEs when their studies indicated that NO plays a role in mediating the contractile function of human and canine prostates.

Mulhall and colleagues[9] assessed the impact of sildenafil on LUTS, using the International Prostate Symptom Scores (IPSS) questionnaire and the International Index of Erectile Function (IIEF). Forty-eight men with IPSS of ≥10 were enrolled in the study and received sildenafil therapy. Baseline scores were recorded, and IIEF and IPSS inventories were repeated at least 3 months after treatment with sildenafil was begun.

The mean improvement in the erectile function score was 7 points ($P$=0.01). The IPSS showed a mean improvement of 4.6 points ($P$=0.013), and the quality-of-life (QOL) score was 1.4 points ($P$=0.025). A total of 60% of the men participating improved their IPSS and 35% had at least a 4-point improvement in their scores, indicating that sildenafil has a positive impact on men with mild-to-moderate LUTS.

A recent study evaluated sildenafil for ED and LUTS in men with both conditions.[10] The study was a 12-week, double-blind, placebo-controlled study of sildenafil in men ≥45 years who scored ≤25 on the erectile function (EF) domain of the IIEF and ≥12 on the IPSS. The primary study outcome was change from baseline in EF assessed using the EF domain of the IIEF. Secondary outcomes were changes from baseline in the other domains of the IIEF, LUTS using the IPSS, QOL score, the BPH Impact Index (B II), peak urinary flow rate ($Q_{max}$), Self-Esteem and Relationship (SEAR) questionnaire scores, and end-of-treatment satisfaction.

Compared with men on placebo, the sildenafil group had greater improvement and higher end-of-treatment scores on the EF domain of the IIEF, meeting the primary outcome objective (Figure 10-1). Sildenafil also met the secondary efficacy objectives for LUTS, showing improvements from baseline comparable with that achieved with α-blockers and 5ARIs, with the exception of changes in $Q_{max}$. The lack of improvement in urinary flow (uroflow) with sildenafil suggests that other pathophysiologic mechanisms may be involved in the etiology of LUTS.

In 11% of patients, headache was the most commonly reported adverse event, followed by dyspepsia (6%), flushing (5%), and rhinitis (4%). One serious adverse event occurred that was possibly related to the study drug: a severe acute cerebrovascular stroke in a 71-year-old man who received 100 mg of sildenafil for 32 days.

Another recent study assessed the efficacy and safety of tadalafil dosed once a day for the treatment of LUTS due to BPH.[11] Eligible patients participated in a 4-week, single-blind, run-in period with placebo prior to treatment with tadalafil. Baseline information was obtained through questionnaires and postvoid residual urine (PVR) volume and uroflowmetry parameters. Patients received either 12 weeks of placebo or 6 weeks of once-a-day dosing with 5 mg tadalafil followed by dose escalation to 20 mg tadalafil for an additional 6 weeks. Primary efficacy end points were IPSS change from baseline to 6 and 12 weeks, and

10

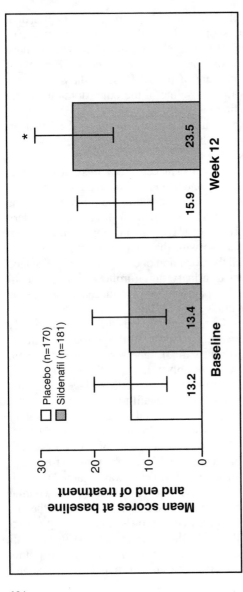

**Figure 10-1:** International Index of Erectile Function (IIEF) baseline and end-of-treatment scores on erectile function domain—sildenafil (Viagra®) vs placebo for ED. Patients completed IIEF domain before treatment and after 12 weeks of either placebo or sildenafil (randomized). Maximum erectile function domain score is 30 points. Higher scores indicate better treatment outcome.

\* Mean change in score from baseline vs placebo change from baseline *P* <0.0001. From McVary et al.[10]

secondary end points assessed additional obstructive and irritative voiding symptoms and QOL.

Compared with placebo, tadalafil showed statistically significant and clinically relevant improvements in LUTS due to BPH. Improvement was observed in both irritative and obstructive symptoms as well as in QOL assessment. Tadalafil treatment, however, did not improve uroflowmetry measures, a finding similar to that reported in a recent sildenafil study.[10] As with the sildenafil study, the lack of improvement in urinary flow (uroflow) may indicate a new mechanism of action. In the subset of LUTS patients who had ED and were sexually active, tadalafil significantly improved erectile function as well as LUTS. The most commonly reported adverse events with tadalafil treatment were 'erection increased,' dyspepsia, back pain, and headache (Table 10-2). No patients discontinued therapy because of 'erection increased,' and no subject reported priapism.

Another recent study by Tinel and associates[12] evaluated the three PDE-5 inhibitors (ie, sildenafil, tadalafil, vardenafil [Levitra®]) for potential efficacy in treating BPH and LUTS. Organ-bath experiments and animal tissue studies showed that the highest expression of PDE-5 mRNA was in the bladder, followed by the urethra and the prostate. Vardenafil was more effective at inhibiting cell proliferation in human prostate stromal cells than were sildenafil and tadalafil. PDE-5 inhibitors induced significant relaxation of the targeted tissues, inhibiting human prostate stromal cell proliferation and reducing the irritative symptoms of LUTS due to BPH. Although more studies are necessary, it appears that PDE-5 inhibitors could be used to effectively treat LUTS due to BPH.

## $\alpha_{1D}$-Adrenergic Receptor Antagonists

The $\alpha$-adrenergic receptor antagonists (or $\alpha$-blockers) were originally developed as antihypertensive drugs, but they are now the most widely used medical therapy for BPH. The dynamic component contributing to BPH is the in-

### Table 10-2: Treatment-Emergent Adverse Events

|  | Placebo 6 wk |  |
|---|---|---|
|  | n=143 |  |
| **TEAE, ≥2% in any treatment group, n (%)** |  |  |
| Erection increased | 2 | (1.4) |
| Dyspepsia | 0 | (0) |
| Back pain | 0 | (0) |
| Headache | 1 | (0.7) |
| Nasopharyngitis | 0 | (0) |
| Upper respiratory tract infection | 1 | (0.7) |
| **Serious adverse events, n (%)** | 0 | (0) |

*Cumulative data reported at 12 weeks.
n=number of patients randomly assigned
TEAE=treatment-emergent adverse events
From McVary et al[11]

crease in smooth muscle tone. The $\alpha_1$-adrenergic receptors are found in the smooth muscle cells of the fibromuscular stromal tissue of the prostate. The $\alpha_1$-adrenergic receptors are stimulated by the neurotransmitter norepinephrine, which mediates the tone of the prostatic smooth muscle. By inhibiting $\alpha_1$-adrenergic receptors, $\alpha$-adrenergic receptor antagonists interrupt the sequence of events. The result is a reduction in prostatic smooth muscle tone, which allows the prostate muscle to relax, which, in turn, diminishes compression of the urethra and facilitates urination.

The $\alpha_1$-adrenergic receptors have been further classified into $\alpha_{1A}$-, $\alpha_{1B}$-, and $\alpha_{1D}$-adrenergic receptor subtypes.

| Tadalafil 5 mg 6 wk | | Placebo* 12 wk | | Tadalafil* 5/20 mg 12 wk | |
|---|---|---|---|---|---|
| n=138 | | n=143 | | n=138 | |
| 5 | (3.6) | 2 | (1.4) | 7 | (5.1) |
| 3 | (2.2) | 0 | (0) | 6 | (4.3) |
| 3 | (2.2) | 2 | (1.4) | 5 | (3.6) |
| 3 | (2.2) | 1 | (0.7) | 4 | (2.9) |
| 2 | (1.4) | 0 | (0) | 3 | (2.2) |
| 2 | (1.4) | 1 | (0.7) | 3 | (2.2) |
| 0 | (0) | 1 | (0.7) | 0 | (0) |

Although $\alpha_1$-adrenergic receptor antagonists terazosin **10** (Hytrin®), doxazosin (Cardura®, Cardura® XL), tamsulosin (Flomax®), and alfuzosin (Uroxatral®) are approved by the FDA for the treatment of LUTS due to BPH, newer agents are in development that may have fewer side effects, be more selective for irritative voiding symptoms, and therefore hold the promise of more efficacy. Two of the investigational $\alpha_1$-adrenergic receptor antagonists in development are naftopidil and silodosin.

### Naftopidil

Animal studies by Ikegaki[13] showed naftopidil to be selective for $\alpha_{1D}$-adrenergic receptor, with approximately

3- and 17-fold higher affinity than for the $\alpha_{1A}$- and $\alpha_{1B}$-adrenergic receptor subtypes, respectively. Naftopidil was found to selectively inhibit phenylephrine-induced prostatic pressure compared with mean blood pressure and was more selective for prostatic pressure than were tamsulosin and prazosin (Minipress®, Minipress® XL). Naftopidil also was shown to have less effect on induced blood pressure reactions than did tamsulosin and prazosin. The study concluded that naftopidil was demonstrated to be effective in the treatment of bladder outlet obstruction (BOO) in patients with BPH.

Two groups of investigators[14,15] examined the effectiveness of naftopidil in 81 patients with LUTS due to BPH. Takahashi and coworkers[14] studied patients who had one or more episodes of urinary urgency/day, a score of ≥8 points on the IPSS, and ≥3 points in any of the scores for three items (urinary frequency, nocturia, and urinary urgency) of the IPSS. The patients received 50 to 75 mg naftopidil/day over 6 weeks. Naftopidil was found to improve not only voiding symptoms but also storage symptoms, and was effective for nocturia in patients with BPH regardless of the existence of nocturnal polyuria (Table 10-3).

Nakatsu and colleagues[15] studied the effect on QOL for 81 patients with BPH due to LUTS. Results were similar to the Takahashi study and indicated that voiding and storage symptoms, total IPSS, QOL index, $Q_{max}$, and PVR volume all showed significant improvement compared with baseline after treatment with naftopidil. Of the 81 patients, two complained of adverse events. The results supported the findings of Takahashi and coworkers that naftopidil is effective for BPH due to LUTS, with improved QOL attributed to improvement in nocturia and incomplete bladder emptying.

In another study, Yamanishi and colleagues[16] examined the efficacy of naftopidil in the treatment of BPH in 49 patients, using the IPSS and urodynamic parameters. Eviprostat, which is a phytotherapeutic agent, was used as a control. In the naftopidil group, the mean total IPSS,

## Table 10-3: Clinical Efficacy of Naftopidil on Overactive Bladder Symptoms in Patients With BPH

|  | IPSS | |
| --- | --- | --- |
|  | *Baseline* | *After 6 Weeks of Therapy** |
| **Total IPSS** | 19.1 points | 10.5 points (*P*<0.0001) |
| **Urgency** | 3.1 | 1.4 (*P*<0.0001) |
| **Frequency:** | | |
| *Daytime* | 9.3 | 8.0 (*P*<0.0001) |
| *Nighttime* | 2.7 | 2.0 (*P*=0.0009) |
| **Mean volume/void** | 174.0 mL | 188.6 mL (*P*=0.0453) |
| **Nocturia** | 3.2 | 2.3 (*P*<0.0001) |
| *Patients <u>with</u> nocturnal polyuria* | | (*P*=0.0006) |
| *Patients <u>without</u> nocturnal polyuria* | | (*P*=0.0135) |

*Naftopidil 50-75 mg/day

BPH=benign prostatic hyperplasia; IPSS=International Prostate Symptom Scores

From Takahashi et al[14]

**10**

voiding symptoms score, and the QOL score all decreased significantly (*P*<0.0001), but there were no significant decrease in those scores in the eviprostat group. The naftopidil group showed significant increases in average uroflow rate, $Q_{max}$, and bladder capacity at first desire to void (*P*<0.0001, *P*=0.0001, and *P*=0.024, respectively). PVR, percentage of residual urine, and the Abrams-Griffiths number also showed significant decreases ($P=0.009$, $P=0.008$, and $P=0.042$, respectively). No significant improvements were seen in the eviprostat group for these parameters. For the pressure-flow study, naftopidil showed a 29% improvement in the International Continence Society nomogram grade vs a 16% improvement for the eviprostat group. Additionally, detrusor overactivity disappeared in 21% of the naftopidil group, whereas cystometric capacity increased in 36%. No improvement was seen in the eviprostat group for detrusor overactivity.

Naftopidil ($\alpha_{1D}$-adrenergic receptor antagonist) was compared with tamsulosin ($\alpha_{1A}$-adrenergic receptor antagonist) for efficacy and safety in the treatment of BPH in a randomized controlled trial by Gotoh and colleagues.[17] Primary variables were changes in the total IPSS, $Q_{max}$, and PVR. The secondary efficacy variables were average uroflow rate, changes in IPSS storage score, IPSS voiding score, and QOL index score over a 12-week period.

Results showed statistically significant improvements from baseline for all primary and secondary variables in both groups, except for PVR in the tamsulosin group; although there was no significant intergroup difference in the improvement of any efficacy variable between the groups. Adverse effects were comparable. The researchers concluded that there was no difference in clinical efficacy or adverse effects between the two $\alpha_1$-adrenergic receptor antagonists, despite different $\alpha_1$ subtypes.

A crossover study by Nishino and coworkers[18] compared naftopidil with tamsulosin for treatment of LUTS due to BPH and arrived at slightly different results. Efficacy criteria were improvement in LUTS by IPSS, QOL score, uroflow-metry, and pressure-flow study values based on treatment with each agent. Naftopidil was significantly more effective than tamsulosin in relieving nocturia. The increases from baseline in the volume at first desire and maximum desire to void were also significantly higher with naftopidil than with tamsulosin. Relief of nocturia may have caused the greater increase in first-desire volume with naftopidil. The decrease in other symptoms of the IPSS, QOL score, increase in uroflowmetry values, and changes in other pressure-flow study values were similar for both agents. This study concluded that naftopidil appeared to be more effective than tamsulosin in the treatment of LUTS due to BPH.

### Silodosin

Silodosin is a novel $\alpha_{1A}$-adrenergic receptor antagonist with a strong affinity for the $\alpha_1$-adrenergic receptor in the human prostate.[19] Studies by Murata and coworkers[20] evaluated the binding and functional affinity of silodosin (KMD-3213) and other $\alpha_1$-adrenergic receptor antagonists, including prazosin and tamsulosin. Silodosin proved as potent as tamsulosin and more potent than prazosin at inhibiting noradrenaline-induced contraction in the human prostate. Importantly, only silodosin showed substantial tissue selectivity, with a more than 100-fold higher affinity for the prostate than for the mesenteric artery.

An animal study[21] assessed the cardiovascular effects of silodosin. Results indicated that the $\alpha_{1A}$-adrenergic receptor subtype was not involved in the regulation of blood pressure, suggesting that the cardiovascular profile of silodosin indicates that it is a safe and well-tolerated drug. Additional in vitro and in vivo studies[22] compared the prostatic selectivity of silodosin with that of other $\alpha_1$-adrenergic receptor antagonists. In vitro, silodosin showed much higher prostatic selectivity (79.4) compared with tamsulosin (1.78), naftopidil (0.55), BMY 7378 (0.115), and prazosin (0.01). In vivo, silodosin dose dependently performed with much less hypotensive effect than either tamsulosin or naftopidil. Silodosin showed a significantly higher uroselectivity (237) than either tamsulosin (1.21) or naftopidil (2.65). Silodosin was shown to be a potent and highly selective $\alpha_{1A}$-adrenergic receptor antagonist with potential as a less hypotensive drug for the treatment of urinary dysfunction in BPH patients.

## Table 10-4: Comparison of Efficacy and Safety of Silodosin vs Tamsulosin and Placebo

| | Score Improvements From Baseline | | |
| | Silodosin | Tamsulosin | Placebo |
|---|---|---|---|
| **Total IPSS** | -8.3 | -6.8 | -5.3 |
| **QOL** | -1.7 | -1.4 | -1.1 |
| **Incidence rates of adverse events and drug-related adverse events** | 88.6%[*] | 82.3% | 71.6% |

[*]Abnormal ejaculation was the most common adverse event in the silodosin group and occurred more often than in the tamsulosin group (22.4% vs 1.6%).

IPSS=International Prostate Symptom Scores; QOL=quality of life

From Kawabe et al[23]

Kawabe and coworkers[23] compared silodosin with tamsulosin in a phase III randomized, placebo-controlled, double-blind study. A total of 457 patients were randomized to silodosin, tamsulosin, and placebo (Table 10-4). Despite the relatively high incidence of abnormal ejaculation in the silodosin group, only 2.9% of the silodosin patients discontinued treatment because of abnormal ejaculation. Silodosin was shown to be clinically useful for treating LUTS due to BPH.

An animal study by Muto and associates[24] evaluated the safety of silodosin. Results showed that silodosin produced

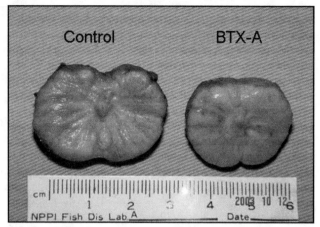

**Figure 10-2:** Coronal section of canine prostate 1 month after botulinum toxin A (BTX-A) or saline injection (control). From Chuang et al.[28]

no severe effects on the central nervous, cardiovascular, or respiratory systems and demonstrated that silodosin had adequate safety margins between the clinically recommended dose and those doses at which toxic effects or safety pharmacologic changes were detected. It appears that silodosin should have few serious side effects in clinical use for the treatment of LUTS due to BPH.

### Botulinum Toxin A Injection for BPH

Intraprostatic injection has been used for more than 100 years as a treatment for BPH[25] and has recently become a subject of renewed interest. Botulinum toxin A (BTX-A) may be an option when medical therapy fails and may also provide an alternative to surgery, which can result in complications and is not always successful.

BTX-A is a neurotoxin that has been successfully used to treat various conditions, including focal dystonias, achalasia, strabismus, and blepharospasm.[26] BTX-A has

## Table 10-5: Patient Profiles and Results After BTX-A Treatment

| Patient | Age (yr) | Prostate Volume (mL) Pre/Post | PSA (ng/mL) Pre/Post | IPSS Pre/Post |
|---------|----------|-------------------------------|----------------------|---------------|
| 1 | 75 | 45.0/40.6 | 4.1/1.6 | 16/2 |
| 2 | 60 | 54.3/40.7 | 4.1/3.2 | 22/15 |
| 3 | 77 | 116.0/85.0 | 9.0/6.6 | 18/13 |
| 4 | 75 | 51.8/36.4 | –/20.7 | 26/2 |
| 5 | 73 | 76.2/61.4 | 4.4 | 25/5 |
| 6 | 70 | 46.3/39.3 | 3.6/- | 11/1 |
| 7 | 72 | 61.8/54.9 | 3.3/3.5 | 19/2 |
| 8 | 67 | 41.3/41.0 | 2.0/2.4 | 15/1 |

– =lack of data

BTX-A=botulinum toxin A; IPSS=International Prostate Symptom Scores; PSA=prostate-specific antigen; $Q_{max}$=peak urinary flow rate

From Chuang et al[29]

also been injected into the bladder or urethra to treat lower urinary tract dysfunction short term (ie, for ≥6 months).

BTX-A blocks the release of neurotransmitters, such as acetylcholine, (ACh) at the neuromuscular junction as well as in autonomic neurons. Intraprostatic injection of BTX-A induces selective denervation and subsequent atrophy of glandular tissue.[27] Unlike some other injectants, such as anhydrous ethanol, BTX-A does not cause localized prostatic necrosis and is a reversible treatment. The effects of denervation wear off in approximately 6 months as new axons develop.[26]

Studies by Chuang and coworkers[28,29] found that BTX-A injection into the prostate alters cellular dynamics by in-

| QOL index Pre/Post | $Q_{max}$ (mL/s) Pre/Post | Postvoid Residual Urine (PVR) (mL) Pre/Post | Follow-up (Month) |
| --- | --- | --- | --- |
| 3/1 | 6/11 | 73/20 | 8 |
| 3/2 | 9.8/13 | 138/20 | 6 |
| 4/2 | 12/14 | 18/15 | 6 |
| 5/1 | 0/12 | 500/24 | 4 |
| 5/2 | 0/12 | 500/40 | 4 |
| 3/1 | 12/15 | 72/17 | 4 |
| 4/2 | 11/14 | 100/48 | 3 |
| 4/1 | 9/12 | 20/12 | 3 |

ducing apoptosis (ie, programmed cell death), inhibiting proliferation, and down-regulating $\alpha_{1A}$-adrenergic receptors. In animal studies, when compared with the control prostate (which was injected with saline), after 1 month of treatment with BTX-A, the canine prostate showed marked atrophy, indicating diffuse apoptosis of prostate glands (Figure 10-2).

In human studies,[28] transperineal injection was performed under transrectal ultrasound guidance. One hundred units of BTX-A were dissolved in 4 mL of 0.9% saline solution, and each lobe of the prostate was injected with 2 mL of BTX-A. Pre- and postoperative evaluations were compared using the

IPSS, QOL scores, $Q_{max}$, PVR volume, and prostate volume. At 1-month follow-up, prostate volume, mean symptom score, and QOL index were significantly reduced by 18%, 73.1%, and 61.5%, respectively. The $Q_{max}$ was increased by 72% and PVR volume decreased by 86.2% (Table 10-5).

Another study[30] evaluated the therapeutic role of BTX-A in men with BPH. Control patients received 4 mL of saline injection, and patients in the treated group received 200 U of BTX-A. No local complications or systemic side effects were observed in any patient. After 2 months, patients receiving BTX-A showed a 65% reduction in AUA symptom scores and a 51% reduction in serum prostate-specific antigen (PSA) levels when compared with baseline. Control patients showed no significant changes in AUA symptom scores or serum PSA levels.

These preliminary studies indicate that BTX-A is a possible effective alternative treatment with minimal adverse effects for patients with BPH for whom medical treatment has failed or who are poor surgical candidates.

## Vitamin D$_3$ Analogues

Calcitriol (1,25-dihydroxyvitamin D$_3$) is the bioactive form of vitamin D. It is a steroid hormone that is synthesized primarily in the kidney and binds to the vitamin D receptor (VDR). VDR agonists have the ability to regulate calcium and bone metabolism and control proliferation and differentiation of various types of cells. By targeting dendritic and T cells, VDR agonists also exhibit anti-inflammatory properties. The prostate is a target organ of VDR agonists and is an extrarenal site for synthesis of calcitriol.[31]

Elocalcitol (BXL-628) is a calcitriol analogue that may offer a new opportunity for the treatment of BPH. Preclinical data demonstrate that VDR agonists, and elocalcitol in particular, reduce prostatic overgrowth by inhibiting the activity of intraprostatic growth factors downstream from the adrenergic receptor. Elocalcitol also targets bladder smooth muscle cells and may reduce irritative bladder symptoms associated with BPH.[31,32] In addition, the anti-inflammatory properties of elocalcitol are likely to have a beneficial effect on the inflammatory component of LUTS.

A phase II clinical study by Colli and colleagues[33] evaluated the effect of elocalcitol on prostate volume in patients with BPH. A total of 119 patients were randomized to receive either elocalcitol 150 μg daily or placebo for 12 weeks. Changes in $Q_{max}$ and American Urological Association Symptom Index (AUA-SI) scores vs baseline were not statistically significant for elocalcitol compared with placebo. However, the percentage change of prostate volume at 12 weeks was significant (-2.90 in the elocalcitol group vs -4.32 in the placebo group [$P<0.0001$]). For men ≥50 years with prostatic volume of ≥40 mL, elocalcitol was able to arrest prostate growth within 12 weeks.

Another study[34] evaluated the effects of elocalcitol on bladder smooth muscle. RhoA/Rho-kinase (ROCK), a calcium-sensitizing pathway, is one of the major intracellular molecules involved in prostatic smooth muscle contraction.[35] An increase in signaling contributes to bladder overactivity through stimulation of bladder smooth muscle.[34] Elocalcitol was shown to impair RhoA membrane translocation and activation and inhibit Rho-kinase activity in bladder smooth muscle. By interrupting this link in bladder smooth muscle stimulation, elocalcitol may be useful in the treatment of altered bladder contractility associated with LUTS due to BPH.

## Metabolic Inhibitors

Metabolic targeting is a new approach to treating disease that takes advantage of the differences in glucose metabolism between normal and diseased cells. Lonidamine (LND) is a derivative of indazole-3-carboxylic acid that has been used safely for more than 20 years in Italy for the treatment of some solid tumors, but the drug is not yet approved for use in the United States.[36] Preliminary data also suggest that LND is effective for the treatment of LUTS due to BPH.

The prostate is primarily an anaerobic organ that depends on glycolysis for energy metabolism.[36-38] The secretory epithelial cells of the peripheral zone (PZ) of the prostate secrete and accumulate high levels of citrate and zinc in the seminal fluid.[37] The high levels of citrate in the prostate inhibit energy production by the Krebs cycle and cause the prostate to be even more dependent on glycolysis. LND is a novel agent that selectively inhibits hexokinase, an essential enzyme that catalyzes glucose, which is the first step in glycolysis.[36,37] By inhibiting hexokinase, LND disrupts energy metabolism in the prostate and causes cell apoptosis.

The efficacy of oral LND treatment in patients with symptomatic BPH was evaluated in an open-label study.[39] Thirty patients received LND 150 mg once daily for 28 days. Subjects were assessed at baseline, 14, and 28 days after initiating therapy, and 1, 2, 3, and 6 months post-treatment for prostate volume, IPSS, $Q_{max}$, PVR, serum PSA levels, serum chemistry, and adverse events.

Patients achieved a significant reduction in prostate volume, increase in $Q_{max}$, decrease in PVR, and reduction in IPSS by day 14 of treatment. However, a large, phase III, randomized, double-blind, placebo-controlled study comparing LND with placebo was recently terminated prematurely because of liver toxicity, and an interim analysis failed to show treatment-dependent symptom improvement.[38]

Metabolic targeting has broad potential applications for both malignant and benign cell proliferation, but further studies are necessary.

## High-Intensity Focused Ultrasound

High-intensity focused ultrasound (HIFU) is a minimally invasive thermal treatment. Although it is not yet available in the United States, it is used for prostate ablation in Europe and other areas of the world. The AUA Guideline for the Treatment of BPH lists HIFU as an emerging therapy for the treatment of BPH.

## Table 10-6: Safety and Effectiveness of Treating BPH With HIFU[*]

| | Center A (20 patients) | Center B (12 patients) | Center C (14 patients) |
|---|---|---|---|
| | % Improvement at 12 Months Compared With Baseline Scores | | |
| **AUA symptom score** | 35% | 43% | 59% |
| **$Q_{max}$** | 30% | 37% | 63% |
| **QOL score** | 63% | ** | 58% |

AUA=American Urological Association; HIFU=high-intensity focused ultrasound; $Q_{max}$=peak urinary flow rate; QOL=quality of life

[*]A total of 46 patients (47 to 84 years) were treated with HIFU at three different centers (A, B, C) with three different protocols.

[**]No figure included.

HIFU is delivered transrectally as opposed to intra-urethrally, so there is no instrumentation or trauma to the urethra. Ideally, HIFU can pinpoint target tissue with precision in a short emission time. The treatment uses concentrated ultrasound energy (0.5 to 10 MHz) that delivers heat ranging between 80° C to 100° C to the targeted tissue, causing tissue ablation. HIFU creates multiple single-focus lesions in the procedure, which lasts approximately 1 hour. Imaging can be performed during the treatment.

A Canadian study by Sullivan and colleagues[40] evaluated the safety and effectiveness of treating BPH with HIFU. Forty-six patients were treated using the Sonablate HIFU device (Focus Surgery, Indianapolis, IN) with three different protocols at three different centers (designated

**Table 10-7: Mean Decrease in IPSS and Mean Increase in $Q_{max}$ in Patients Who Did Not Require a Secondary Procedure After Treatment for BPH**

|        | IPSS  | $Q_{max}$ (mL/s) |
|--------|-------|------------------|
| **TURP** | -13.9 | +11.5 |
| **TUVP** | -12.7 | +11.1 |
| **VLAP** | -12.9 | +5.6  |
| **HIFU** | -7.0  | +2.5  |
| **TUNA** | -9.8  | +2.3  |

IPSS=International Prostate Symptom Scores; $Q_{max}$=peak urinary flow rate; TUNA=transurethral needle ablation; TURP=transurethral resection of the prostate; UVP=transurethral electrovaporization of the prostate; VLAP=visual laser ablation of the prostate

From Schatzl et al[41]

here as A, B, and C). Baseline and outcome measures were compared for AUA symptom score, $Q_{max}$, and QOL score, and all parameters showed improvements at 12 months post-treatment (Table 10-6).

Complications included hematospermia (13%), perineal pain (11%), mild-to-moderate hematuria (9%), epididymitis (9%), and urinary retention (4%). Recatheterization was necessary in up to 16% of patients, and 11 patients in groups A and B required a TURP because of urinary obstruction after HIFU. No patients in the C group required a TURP. The investigators concluded that HIFU is safe, produces acceptable complications, and effectively relieves BPH symptoms.

In a French study, the clinical literature on HIFU was reviewed by Chartier-Kastler and coworkers.[42] The study found that the quality of ultrasound detection of the target limits the usefulness of HIFU. Optimal firing parameters are necessary for good therapeutic effect on the target tissue while sparing intervening tissue.

An Austrian study by Schatzl and colleagues[41] compared the effectiveness of TURP with four less invasive therapeutic options during a 2-year follow-up. Ninety-five elderly men were assigned prospectively to one of five treatment arms: 28 to TURP, 17 to transurethral electrovaporization of the prostate (TUVP), 17 to visual laser ablation of the prostate (VLAP), 20 to HIFU, and 15 to transurethral needle ablation (TUNA) of the prostate. IPSS, $Q_{max}$, and uroflowmetry were assessed at 6, 12, 18, and 24 months postoperatively. During the study, one patient (4%) in the TURP group required a secondary TURP, four (23.5%) needed a TURP after TUVP, four (26.7%) needed a TURP after VLAP, four (15%) needed a TURP after HIFU, and three needed a TURP (20%) after TUNA. Table 10-7 compares the mean decrease in IPSS and mean increase in $Q_{max}$ in patients who did not require a secondary procedure.

In a long-term analysis of 80 men with LUTS due to BPH who underwent HIFU,[43] patients were evaluated every 6 months for 4 years after treatment. Although American Urological Association-International Prostate Symptom Scores (AUA-IPSS) decreased 53%, from 19.6 preoperatively to 8.5 after 12 months of treatment and remained relatively stable during the 4-year study period, $Q_{max}$ increased from 9.1 mL/sec preoperatively to 11.8 mL/sec after 12 months then gradually declined to 10.2 mL/sec over 4 years. A significant finding was that 35 men (43.8%) underwent TURP during the 4-year study period because of a poor therapeutic response to HIFU treatment. The mean time interval between HIFU treatment and TURP was 26.5 +/- 2.7 months. Further clinical trials are needed for validation of HIFU as an effective treatment for BPH.

10

# References

1. Schwinn DA: The role of alpha 1-adrenergic receptor subtypes in lower urinary tract symptoms. *BJU Int* 2001;88(suppl 2):26-34 (discussion 49-50).

2. Issa MM, Marshall FF: Medical management of benign prostatic hyperplasia. In: *Contemporary Diagnosis and Management of Diseases of the Prostate*, 3rd ed. Newtown, PA, Handbooks in Health Care Co, 2005, pp 54-71.

3. McConnell J, Roehrborn C, Bautista O, et al: The long-term effect of doxazosin, finasteride, and combination therapy on the clinical progression of benign prostatic hyperplasia. *N Engl J Med* 2003;349:2387-2398.

4. Roehrborn CG, Boyle P, Nickel JC, et al: Efficacy and safety of a dual inhibitor of 5-alpha-reductase types 1 and 2 (dutasteride) in men with benign prostatic hyperplasia. *Urology* 2002;60:434-441.

5. Roehrborn C, McConnell J: Etiology, pathophysiology, epidemiology, and natural history of benign prostatic hyperplasia. In: Walsh P, Retik A, Vaughan E, et al, eds: *Campbell's Urology*, 8th ed. Philadelphia, PA, WB Saunders Co, 2002, pp 1297-1336.

6. Johannes CB, Araujo AB, Feldman HA, et al: Incidence of erectile dysfunction in men 40 to 69 years old: longitudinal results from the Massachusetts male aging study. *J Urol* 2000;163:460-463.

7. Roehrborn CG: Lower urinary tract symptoms, benign prostatic hyperplasia, erectile dysfunction, and phosphodiesterase-5 inhibitors. *Rev Urol* 2004;6:121-127.

8. Takeda M, Tang R, Shapiro E, et al: Effects of nitric oxide on human and canine prostates. *Urology* 1995;45:440-446.

9. Mulhall JP, Guhring P, Parker M, et al: Assessment of the impact of sildenafil citrate on lower urinary tract symptoms in men with erectile dysfunction. *J Sex Med* 2006;3:662-667.

10. McVary KT, Monnig W, Camps JL, et al: Sildenafil citrate improves erectile function and urinary symptoms in men with erectile dysfunction and lower urinary tract symptoms associated with benign prostatic hyperplasia: a randomized, double-blind trial. *J Urol* 2007;177:1071-1077.

11. McVary KT, Roehrborn CG, Kaminetsky JC, et al: Tadalafil relieves lower urinary tract symptoms secondary to benign prostatic hyperplasia. *J Urol* 2007;177:1401-1407.

12. Tinel H, Stelte-Ludwig B, Hutter J, et al: Pre-clinical evidence for the use of phosphodiesterase-5 inhibitors for treating benign prostatic hyperplasia and lower urinary tract symptoms. *BJU Int* 2006;98:1259-1263.

13. Ikegaki I: [Pharmacological properties of naftopidil, a drug for treatment of the bladder outlet obstruction for patients with benign prostatic hyperplasia]. *Nippon Yakurigaku Zasshi* 2000;116:63-69.

14. Takahashi S, Tajima A, Matsushima H, et al: Clinical efficacy of an alpha1A/D-adrenoceptor blocker (naftopidil) on overactive bladder symptoms in patients with benign prostatic hyperplasia. *Int J Urol* 2006;13:15-20.

15. Nakatsu H, Naoi M, Sekiyama K, et al: [The effectiveness of naftopidil in patients with benign prostatic hyperplasia evaluated by QOL index]. *Hinyokika Kiyo* 2007;53:13-18.

16. Yamanishi T, Yasuda K, Kamai T, et al: Single-blind, randomized controlled study of the clinical and urodynamic effects of an alpha-blocker (naftopidil) and phytotherapy (eviprostat) in the treatment of benign prostatic hyperplasia. *Int J Urol* 2004;11:501-509.

17. Gotoh M, Kamihira O, Kinukawa T, et al: Comparison of tamsulosin and naftopidil for efficacy and safety in the treatment of benign prostatic hyperplasia: a randomized controlled trial. *BJU Int* 2005;96:581-586.

18. Nishino Y, Masue T, Miwa K, et al: Comparison of two alpha1-adrenoceptor antagonists, naftopidil and tamsulosin hydrochloride, in the treatment of lower urinary tract symptoms with benign prostatic hyperplasia: a randomized crossover study. *BJU Int* 2006;97:747-751.

19. Moriyama N, Akiyama K, Murata S, et al: KMD-3213, a novel alpha1A-adrenoceptor antagonist, potently inhibits the functional alpha1-adrenoceptor in human prostate. *Eur J Pharmacol* 1997;331:39-42.

20. Murata S, Taniguchi T, Takahashi S, et al: Tissue selectivity of KMD-3213, an alpha(1)-adrenoceptor antagonist, in human prostate and vasculature. *J Urol* 2000;164:578-583.

21. Tatemichi S, Kiguchi S, Kobayashi M, et al: Cardiovascular effects of the selective alpha1A-adrenoceptor antagonist silodosin (KMD-3213), a drug for the treatment of voiding dysfunction. *Arzneimittelforschung* 2006;56:682-687.

213

22. Tatemichi S, Tomiyama Y, Maruyama I, et al: Uroselectivity in male dogs of silodosin (KMD-3213), a novel drug for the obstructive component of benign prostatic hyperplasia. *Neurourol Urodyn* 2006;25:792-799.

23. Kawabe K, Yoshida M, Homma Y, et al: Silodosin, a new alpha1A-adrenoceptor-selective antagonist for treating benign prostatic hyperplasia: results of a phase III randomized, placebo-controlled, double-blind study in Japanese men. *BJU Int* 2006;98:1019-1024.

24. Muto S, Kasahara H, Yokoi R, et al: [Toxicity profile of silodosin (KMD-3213)]. *Yakugaku Zasshi* 2006;126:247-256.

25. Plante MK, Folsom JB, Zvara P: Prostatic tissue ablation by injection: a literature review. *J Urol* 2004;172:20-26.

26. Smith CP, Chancellor MB: Emerging role of botulinum toxin in the management of voiding dysfunction. *J Urol* 2004;171:2128-2137.

27. Doggweiler R, Zermann DH, Ishigooka M, et al: Botox-induced prostatic involution. *Prostate* 1998;37:44-50.

28. Chuang YC, Tu CH, Huang CC, et al: Intraprostatic injection of botulinum toxin type-A relieves bladder outlet obstruction in human and induces prostate apoptosis in dogs. *BMC Urol* 2006;6:12.

29. Chuang YC, Huang CC, Kang HY, et al: Novel action of botulinum toxin on the stromal and epithelial components of the prostate gland. *J Urol* 2006;175(3 pt 1):1158-1163.

30. Maria G, Brisinda G, Civello IM, et al: Relief by botulinum toxin of voiding dysfunction due to benign prostatic hyperplasia: results of a randomized, placebo-controlled study. *Urology* 2003;62:259-264; discussion 264-265.

31. Maggi M, Crescioli C, Morelli A, et al: Pre-clinical evidence and clinical translation of benign prostatic hyperplasia treatment by the vitamin D receptor agonist BXL-628 (Elocalcitol). *J Endocrinol Invest* 2006;29:665-674.

32. Adorini L, Penna G, Amuchastegui S, et al: Inhibition of prostate growth and inflammation by the vitamin D receptor agonist BXL-628 (elocalcitol). *J Steroid Biochem Mol Biol* 2007;103:689-693.

33. Colli E, Rigatti P, Montorsi F, et al: BXL628, a novel vitamin D3 analog arrests prostate growth in patients with benign prostatic hyperplasia: a randomized clinical trial. *Eur Urol* 2006;49:82-86.

34. Morelli A, Vignozzi L, Filippi S, et al: BXL-628, a vitamin D receptor agonist effective in benign prostatic hyperplasia treatment, prevents RhoA activation and inhibits RhoA/Rho kinase signaling in rat and human bladder. *Prostate* 2007;67:234-247.

35. Takahashi R, Nishimura J, Seki N, et al: RhoA/Rho kinase-mediated Ca(2+) sensitization in the contraction of human prostate. *Neurourol Urodyn* 2007;26:547-551.

36. Roehrborn CG: The development of lonidamine for benign prostatic hyperplasia and other indications. *Rev Urol* 2005;7(suppl 7): S12-S20.

37. Costello LC, Franklin RB: The clinical relevance of the metabolism of prostate cancer; zinc and tumor suppression: connecting the dots. *Mol Cancer* 2006;15;5:17.

38. Lepor H: The role of gonadotropin-releasing hormone antagonists for the treatment of benign prostatic hyperplasia. *Rev Urol* 2006;8:183-189.

39. Ditonno P, Battaglia M, Selvaggio O, et al: Clinical evidence supporting the role of lonidamine for the treatment of BPH. *Rev Urol* 2005;7(suppl 7):S27-S33.

40. Sullivan L, Casey RW, Pommerville PJ, et al: Canadian experience with high intensity focused ultrasound for the treatment of BPH. *Can J Urol* 1999;6:799-805.

41. Schatzl G, Madersbacher S, Djavan B, et al: Two-year results of transurethral resection of the prostate versus four 'less invasive' treatment options. *Eur Urol* 2000;37:695-701.

42. Chartier-Kastler E, Yonneau L, Conort P, et al: [High-intensity focused ultrasound (HIFU) in urology]. *Prog Urol* 2000;10:1108-1117.

43. Madersbacher S, Schatzl G, Djavan B, et al: Long-term outcome of transrectal high-intensity focused ultrasound therapy for benign prostatic hyperplasia. *Eur Urol* 2000;37:687-694.

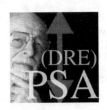

# 20 Most Frequently Asked Questions About BPH

**1. What is the natural history of benign prostatic hyperplasia (BPH) if left untreated? What percentage of men would have increased symptoms?**

**A.** BPH is a progressive disease that begins to develop histologically as early as the age of 25 to 30 in some men[1] and is identifiable histologically in approximately 90% of men in their 90s.[2] The likelihood of progression of lower urinary tract symptoms (LUTS) due to BPH appears to depend on the initial severity of symptoms, with measurable progression in symptom severity over 3.5 to 4 years (Olmsted County Study of Urinary Symptoms and Health Status Among Men). The study showed that men with mild urinary symptoms initially (67%) experienced worsened symptoms over a 4-year period (50% progressed to moderate symptoms, 7% to severe symptoms, and 10% chose surgery). Men with moderate symptoms initially (41%) progressed to severe symptoms, and 24% underwent surgery. Patients with severe symptoms at the initial time of observation (39%) chose surgery over a 4-year period.[3]

**2. When should 5α-reductase inhibitors (5ARIs) be used as monotherapy?**

**A.** For patients who have a large prostate, but mild or no symptoms, use of a 5ARI, such as dutasteride (Avodart®)

or finasteride (Proscar®), is suggested. The rationale is that a 5ARI will shrink the prostate and retard further growth, which will reduce the risk of urinary retention and surgery in the future. Use of a single agent also keeps adverse side effects to a minimum.

### 3. How does a 5ARI (eg, dutasteride) affect prostate-specific antigen (PSA) values and/or screening for prostate cancer?

**A.** Treatment with a 5ARI, such as dutasteride, decreases PSA levels by approximately 50% over 4 to 6 months.[4-6] Because serum PSA level plays a role in screening for prostate cancer, and BPH and prostate cancer can be present in the same patient, it is important to be able to calculate the PSA value in men taking dutasteride. Osterling et al[7] suggest that mathematically doubling the serum PSA level provides an approximation for interpretation of PSA for cancer detection in finasteride-treated patients. Sustained increases in PSA during dutasteride or finasteride treatment, however, should be carefully evaluated with a prostate biopsy.

### 4. What are the indications for open prostatectomy as a treatment for BPH?

**A.** A relatively invasive procedure that is associated with comorbidities, open prostatectomy is now reserved for men with large prostates (ie, >70 to 100 g) and symptomatic BPH, with or without concomitant bladder pathologies, such as diverticula or bladder calculi. Open prostatectomy provides a definitive and effective long-term treatment, but it is associated with a relatively long hospitalization time (ie, 2 to 4 days), greater perioperative blood loss than alternative procedures, and a longer recuperative period. Open prostatectomy is seldom performed in the United States today, comprising <3% of surgical procedures performed for BPH management.[8] The expected results and risks involved should be carefully evaluated by the surgeon and the patient.

## 5. What is the relationship between BPH and erectile dysfunction (ED)? Is there any overlap in their medical management?

**A.** Emerging evidence indicates a strong link between BPH and ED.[9] Patients with LUTS frequently also have ED, and those with ED frequently experience LUTS.

Nerve terminals release the neurotransmitter nitric oxide (NO), which is involved in the relaxation of the corpus cavernosum smooth muscle and vasculature of the penis. Aging, diabetes, hypertension, and smoking are among the conditions that are associated with reduced function of nerves and endothelium and are also conditions that are associated with ED. A decrease in production of NO within the prostate and erectile tissues may, therefore, manifest as ED and LUTS comorbidities. Additional theories linking ED and LUTS include prostate and penile ischemia, Rho-kinase activation activity, and autonomic hyperactivity, which, in turn, affect LUTS, prostate growth, and ED.[10]

Phosphodiesterase-5 (PDE-5) inhibitors are approved for use in treating ED, and preliminary studies on all three PDE-5 inhibitors (ie, sildenafil [Revatio™, Viagra®], tadalafil [Cialis®], vardenafil [Levitra®]) indicate they could also be used effectively to treat LUTS due to BPH.[11-13]

## 6. How do you work up a patient who presents to your office with symptoms related to BPH?

**A.** *History:* An initial history should rule out other possible causes of obstructed urinary flow (uroflow) (ie, neurologic disorders, urinary tract infection [UTI], bladder or prostate neoplasms, urethral stricture or injury, prostatitis, neurogenic bladder), and inquiries should be made about previous urinary tract problems and hematuria. The patient's medications should be reviewed for use of anticholinergics (antihistamines) and sympathomimetics (decongestants), which can contribute to urinary problems.

*Questionnaires:* The American Urological Association Symptom Index (AUA-SI) and BPH Impact Index (B II) help assess the severity of symptoms and the degree of bother, respectively. In addition, the nine-question International Index of Erectile Function (IIEF) will help assess ED and the Male Sexual Health Questionnaire to Assess Ejaculatory Dysfunction (MSHQ-EjD short form) can be used to evaluate ejaculatory dysfunction.

*Physical Examination:* A digital rectal examination (DRE) and assessment of anal sphincter tone should be performed to help evaluate prostate size. The bladder should be palpated, and the lower extremities assessed for edema, peripheral pulses, and neurologic reflexes.

*Tests:* A urinalysis and serum PSA test should be performed routinely for every patient with LUTS. Additional tests, including serum creatinine, renal ultrasonography, uroflowmetry, urine cytology, and cystoscopy, are appropriate for specific concerns but are not routine tests. For evaluating patients with complicating conditions, see Chapter 3.

*Voiding Diary:* A voiding diary is a simple and inexpensive means to assess if lifestyle issues or excessive fluid intake are affecting LUTS. The diary is especially useful for patients with the complaint of nocturia.

*Algorithm:* Figure 3-3 is a useful tool for the initial assessment and diagnosis of LUTS due to BPH.

## 7. What are some of the proposed causes (ie, pathologic mechanisms) of BPH?

**A.** The etiology of BPH continues to be elusive, but aging and normal testicular function appear to be essential components for the development of BPH. There are four main hypotheses regarding the etiology of BPH: the dihydrotestosterone (DHT) or altered hormone environment hypothesis, the embryonic reawakening hypothesis, the stem cell hypothesis, and the nonandrogenic testis factor (NATF) hypothesis.

DHT, which is converted from the androgenic hormone testosterone, is responsible for growth and maintenance of the normal mature prostate.[14,15] An altered hormone environment is one hypothesis for the etiology of BPH. In addition to androgens, the testes produce estrogen, which increases with age while testosterone production decreases. Estrogen increases the amount of androgen receptor in the prostate, increasing androgen-mediated growth, even as testosterone production diminishes.[16]

The embryonic reawakening hypothesis is based on the fact that factors released by stromal prostatic cells influence proliferation, differentiation, and cell death of adjacent epithelial cells,[17,18] and conversely, factors released by epithelial prostatic cells affect stromal prostatic cell proliferation and function.[19] These cells undergo a growth spurt similar to embryonic development, using the same growth mechanisms.

The stem cell hypothesis refers to the fact that, if stem cells are blocked from undergoing apoptosis (ie, normal cell death), prostatic overgrowth may occur.[20]

The NATF hypothesis proposes that the testes secrete a nonandrogenic prostate growth-stimulating factor, almost certainly a protein, that plays a critical role in the ubiquitous development of histologic BPH and possibly a contributory role in the subsequent development of mass-producing BPH.[21,22]

### 8. Does BPH cause prostate cancer? How does PSA correlate with BPH?

**A.** BPH and prostate cancer can exist concomitantly, but BPH does not cause cancer. The transition zone (TZ) of the prostate gland—specifically the periurethral portion of the TZ—is where nonmalignant proliferation (BPH) occurs. Most prostate cancers develop in the peripheral zone (PZ) of the prostate.[23,24]

The prostate secretes PSA, and PSA levels rise with an increase in prostate volume (ie, BPH, prostate cancer). Prostate cancer should be ruled out in the initial evaluation for a patient with LUTS and an increased PSA level.

Serum PSA and prostate volume are closely related. Serum PSA values >1.3 ng/mL at baseline evaluation are associated with an increased risk of BPH progression including increased bothersome LUTS, reduced uroflow rate, faster symptom deterioration, and an impaired quality of life (QOL).[25,26]

High serum PSA in patients with BPH has also been associated with an increased risk of acute urinary retention (AUR) and BPH-related surgery.[27,28] PSA levels greater than age-appropriate norms, an increase in PSA >75 ng/dL/ year, or a PSA >4 ng/mL indicate the need for a prostate biopsy or a repeat PSA test.

### 9. If a patient has many medical conditions and is not medically fit for surgery, can he still undergo treatment for LUTS due to BPH?

**A.** Men who have BPH and many medical conditions and who are not medically fit for surgical treatment still have treatment options for their LUTS.

When coronary artery disease is concomitant with BPH, combined $\alpha_{1A}$- and $\alpha_{1D}$-receptor antagonist action is a good option for treatment. Newer generation pharmaceuticals that specifically bind $\alpha_{1A}$-subtypes, which minimize vascular side effects, such as hypotension, mediated by $\alpha_{1D}$-subtypes, may be appropriate for men with BPH who have comorbidities and who are not medically fit for surgery. Tamsulosin (Flomax®) is a third-generation $\alpha_1$-adrenergic antagonist that selectively targets the smooth muscle cells of the prostate while exerting minimal effects on other $\alpha$-adrenergic receptor subtypes that regulate blood pressure and vasodilatation. It can be coadministered with antihypertensive medications without increasing the risk of hypotensive or syncopal episodes,[29,30] and may, therefore, be useful for BPH patients with cardiovascular disease.

Similarly, alfuzosin (in the extended-release formulation, Uroxatral®) has a high-technology pill matrix structure that allows for a gradual release of the drug. This slow release results in a reduced risk of cardiovascular side effects. Thus this medication can also be used in an at-risk population.

Combining a hormonal agent with an α-adrenergic antagonist has been shown to reduce the risk of BPH progression (Medical Therapy of Prostatic Symptoms [MTOPS] study) and may also be an option for BPH patients who are not medically fit for surgery.

Prostatic stents were developed as an alternative minimally invasive treatment (MIT) to provide relief for prostatic obstruction. Permanent stents are an option for elderly men with significant comorbidities who are medically unfit for surgery. However, one study[31] showed a failure rate of about 25% for permanent stents, and another recent study found that only 37% of stents remained in situ after 6 months and 78% had been removed by 2 years after placement. These statistics support the finding that stents should only be used as an alternative to catheterization in high-risk patients presenting with recurrent urinary retention and who are unfit for surgery.

High-risk patients can also be treated with MITs, such as transurethral microwave thermotherapy (TUMT) and transurethral needle ablation (TUNA), because these treatments are performed with local anesthesia only.

### 10. What evidence suggests that saw palmetto (Serenoa repens) has efficacy in the treatment of BPH?

**A.** Although the exact mechanism of action for saw palmetto is unclear, several questionable lines of evidence indicate that use of the extract from saw palmetto may have a limited effect for the treatment of LUTS due to BPH. Several poorly designed studies comparing saw palmetto to alfuzosin, finasteride, and tamsulosin suggest that saw palmetto may have modest efficacy (at most) in increasing peak urinary flow rate ($Q_{max}$).[32,33] When rigorously studied in patients followed for 1 year, saw palmetto fails to improve the signs and symptoms of LUTS due to BPH. It is not clear if a longer treatment duration or higher doses will improve this therapy. When used to treat BPH, saw palmetto has shown a low frequency of side effects.

### 11. What are the symptoms related to urinary obstruction from an enlarged prostate (EP)?

**A.** An EP that compresses the urethra and compromises uroflow causes bladder outlet obstruction (BOO). Obstructive voiding symptoms include weak stream, hesitancy, straining to void, and incomplete bladder emptying.

### 12. What is the connection between BPH and the metabolic syndrome?

**A.** There are strong connections between BPH and the metabolic syndrome. Results from the Third National Health and Nutrition Examination Study (NHANES III) indicate that a history of diabetes mellitus and hypertension as well as elevated glycosylated hemoglobin are all associated with the presence of LUTS.[34] Abdominal obesity (as measured by waist circumference) and elevated serum insulin levels were significantly associated with increased risk of BPH in a study by Dahle et al.[35] A study of black men found an association between LUTS and type 2 diabetes, hypertension, and cardiovascular disease.[36] Other studies demonstrated that such measures of the metabolic syndrome as elevated body mass index (BMI), waist circumference, dyslipidemia, and fasting plasma insulin levels were related to an increase in annual prostate growth, as were noninsulin-dependent diabetes and hypertension.[37,38]

Proposed etiologies linking the metabolic syndrome and LUTS include changes attributed to chronic, low-grade inflammation, sympathetic nervous system and hormonal changes, and the direct effects of hyperinsulinemia. Autonomic neuropathy associated with diabetes mellitus can affect bladder contractility and lead to voiding dysfunction, and elevated blood-glucose levels can lead to polyuria and nocturia.

### 13. What zone of the prostate typically harbors BPH? Is this different than the zone where prostate cancer arises?

**A.** The innermost part of the prostate gland where it wraps around the urethra is the TZ, and the periurethral portion of

FAQs

the TZ is the primary site where BPH develops. Prostate cancer rarely (ie, approximately 10%) develops in the TZ. The PZ, which is at the back of the prostate close to the rectum, is where most prostate cancer develops.

### 14. Are there any benefits to combined medical therapy with a 5ARI and an α-adrenergic antagonist?

**A.** Because 5ARIs target the static component of BPH, and α-adrenergic therapy affects the dynamic component of BPH, a combination of the two theoretically should provide the benefits of each medication. The MTOPS study[39,40] demonstrated that combination therapy resulted in a significant risk reduction in the progression of BPH compared with monotherapy. Findings included a sustained measurable decrease in American Urological Association-International Prostate Symptom Scores (AUA-IPSS) and a decreased risk of developing AUR or undergoing surgery for treatment of BPH.

When taking combination therapy, adverse events are similar to those for each drug alone. Several adverse events, however, were increased in those taking combination therapy—abnormal ejaculation, peripheral edema, and dyspnea.[40]

### 15. Are there differences in the outcomes (as measured by retreatment rate, need for continued medical therapy) for open prostatectomy, transurethral resection of the prostate (TURP), and the newer MITs?

**A.** Outcomes differ in terms of retreatment rates and need for continued medical therapy after open prostatectomy, TURP, and MITs.

A recent prospective study[41] of 56 patients who received an 11-year postoperative follow-up reported that all patients experienced significant decreases in their AUA-SI and QOL scores. Importantly, <2% of patients required continued medication for symptom management after treatment. Despite a risk of a greater perioperative blood loss compared with other procedures, open prostatectomy results in lasting symptomatic improvement with a rare need for further medical therapy or surgical treatment.

TURP is associated with some complications and comorbidities including intraoperative problems, such as bleeding; transurethral resection (TUR) syndrome; cardiovascular disorders; and perforation, as well as postoperative disorders, such as urethral stricture and bladder neck contracture. The rate of retreatment (either medical or surgical) is as high as 20%,[42] with approximately 5% of patients requiring surgical intervention for recurring LUTS due to BPH over a 3-year period following TURP.[43,44]

Transurethral electrovaporization of the prostate (TUVP) is a modification of TURP in which prostatic tissue is vaporized instead of being cut into pieces and removed. Treatment failure requiring a reoperation for BPH-related LUTS or urinary retention occurs in 4% to 7% of patients within the first postoperative year.[45]

Among the MITs for BPH, one study reported that transurethral microwave thermotherapy (TUMT) had a retreatment rate due to recurring LUTS of about 25% during a 3-year follow-up period.[46] Another study showed that after just 2 years, 46.9% of patients were using medical therapy with an $\alpha$-adrenergic antagonist and 17.6% of patients chose to undergo TURP.[47] However, compared with TURP, TUMT is associated with significantly lower postoperative frequencies of urinary incontinence, bladder neck contractures, and urethral strictures.[42,45,48,49]

Similar to TUMT, TUNA is associated with up to 25% retreatment within 3 years due to treatment failure and almost 30% within 5 years. Also similar to TUMT, the overall incidence of postoperative complications is significantly lower than with TURP.[50]

The use of prostatic stents is controversial, and efficacy is variable, depending upon the stent used. Permanent stents have shown a long-term failure rate of approximately 25%.[51] It is recommended that permanent stents only be used as an alternative to catheterization in high-risk patients who are unfit for surgery and who have recurrent urinary retention.[52]

Water-induced thermotherapy (WIT) is a technology that requires additional clinical studies to evaluate its efficacy and morbidities. Some studies report the need for a secondary treatment rate of approximately 5% to 6% at 1-year post-procedure.[53] Adverse outcomes following WIT are similar to other MITs, and AUR occurs in 10% to 15% of patients after WIT, requiring recatheterization.

### 16. What is TUR syndrome?

**A.** When an excessive amount of the glycine irrigation fluid used during TURP (or TUVP) is absorbed into the circulatory system, a clinical syndrome called TUR syndrome develops. The excess fluid results in hypervolemia, hyponatremia, and hyperammonemia. Clinical manifestations of this syndrome include confusion, nausea, vomiting, visual disturbances, bradycardia, and hypertension.[54,55] The incidence of TUR syndrome ranges from 1% to 7%, and the risk of TUR syndrome increases for surgeries lasting >90 minutes and for prostates >35 g.[56]

As soon as TUR syndrome is recognized, the procedure should be terminated. Treatment includes diuretics and sometimes hypertonic saline. Use of bipolar high-frequency current for TURP is a recent technologic development that allows the use of 0.9% saline chloride as the irrigant instead of glycine. Phase III trials indicate the bipolar device may offer some advantages in the reduction of TUR syndrome.[57] TUR syndrome does not occur with holmium laser resection of the prostate (HoLRP), holmium laser enucleation of the prostate (HoLEP), or interstitial laser coagulation (ILC).

### 17. What are the consequences of BPH if left untreated?

**A.** Untreated BPH can lead to a range of complications including AUR, BPH-related surgery, urinary incontinence, hematuria, UTIs, bladder calculi, bladder decompensation, and renal failure. Death may even result from the complications of untreated BPH.[58]

### 18. What should you do if a patient has persistent urinary tract symptoms after undergoing surgical treatment for BPH?

**A.** Persistent urinary tract symptoms after surgery for BPH require re-evaluation, usually by endoscopic, voiding cystourethorography, and/or urodynamic studies. Residual obstructive tissue may be the cause or other factors, including a previously unidentified neurogenic dysfunction, may be the cause. Unresolved urinary tract symptoms may require reoperation.

### 19. What are the indications for surgical treatment for BPH?

**A.** Absolute indications for surgical treatment of BPH include moderate-to-severe LUTS (AUA-SI ≥8), bladder calculi, renal insufficiency, AUR, recurrent UTIs, and renal failure due to BOO. In addition, patients who have failed medical therapy or prefer a one-time method of treatment for their LUTS may choose surgery over medical management. All factors should be weighed before the patient and physician make a decision to initiate surgical treatment for BPH.

### 20. Is BPH a rare condition? What are the risk factors for BPH?

**A.** BPH is the most common nonmalignant disorder of the prostate and the most common tumor in men >60 years.[59] The incidence of BPH increases with age. Anatomic or microscopic BPH is present in 20% of men ages 40 to 50, 40% of men 50 to 60, 55% of men 60 to 70, 80% of men 70 to 80, and 90% of men 80 to 90 years of age.[59] Approximately 30% of white American men >50 years have moderate-to-severe LUTS due to BPH.[60,61]

The presence of androgens is essential for the development of BPH, and aging is a major risk factor. Studies have indicated a positive association with a family history of BPH, resulting in the development of BPH-related symptoms at an earlier age (ie, <60 years).[59,62,63] Geographic location appears to have a negligible impact on the risk of developing BPH, but race and ethnicity do have an effect on the probability of developing BPH, with black and Hispanic men at a 41% higher risk for total BPH than white men.[64] Several studies report an inverse relationship between BMI and BPH, with a reduced risk of BPH as BMI increases.[65-67] One theory for this phenomenon is that adipose tissue is one of the major sites where androgens are converted into estrogens, resulting in lower serum testosterone.

## References

1. McNeal JE, Redwine EA, Freiha FS, et al: Zonal distribution of prostatic adenocarcinoma. Correlation with histologic pattern and direction of spread. *Am J Surg Pathol* 1988;12:897-906.

2. Harbitz TB, Haugen OA: Histology of the prostate in elderly men. A study in an autopsy series. *Acta Pathol Microbiol Scand [A]* 1972;80:756-768.

3. Guess HA, Jacobsen SJ, Girman CJ, et al: The role of community-based longitudinal studies in evaluating treatment effects. Example: benign prostatic hyperplasia. *Med Care* 1995;33(4 suppl): AS26-AS35.

4. Guess HA, Heyse JF, Gormley GJ: The effect of finasteride on prostate-specific antigen in men with benign prostatic hyperplasia. *Prostate* 1993;22:31-37.

5. Guess HA, Heyse JF, Gormley GJ, et al: Effect of finasteride on serum PSA concentration in men with benign prostatic hyperplasia. Results from the North American phase III clinical trial. *Urol Clin North Am* 1993;20:627-636.

6. Lange PH: Is the prostate pill finally here? *N Engl J Med* 1992; 327:1234-1236.

7. Oesterling JE, Roy J, Agha A, et al: Biologic variability of prostate-specific antigen and its usefulness as a marker for prostate cancer: effects of finasteride. The Finasteride PSA Study Group. *Urology* 1997;50:13-18.

8. Bruskewitz R: Management of symptomatic BPH in the US: who is treated and how? *Eur Urol* 1999;36(suppl 3):7-13.

9. McVary K: Lower urinary tract symptoms and sexual dysfunction: epidemiology and pathophysiology. *BJU Int* 2006;97(suppl 2):23-28; discussion 44-45.

10.  McVary KT: Erectile dysfunction and lower urinary tract symptoms secondary to BPH. *Eur Urol* 2005;47:838-845.

11.  McVary KT, Monnig W, Camps JL, et al: Sildenafil citrate improves erectile function and urinary symptoms in men with erectile dysfunction and lower urinary tract symptoms associated with benign prostatic hyperplasia: a randomized, double-blind trial. *J Urol* 2007;177:1071-1077.

12.  McVary KT, Roehrborn CG, Kaminetsky JC, et al: Tadalafil relieves lower urinary tract symptoms (LUTS) secondary to benign prostatic hyperplasia (BPH). *J Urol* 2007;177:1401-1407.

13.  Tinel H, Stelte-Ludwig B, Hutter J, et al: Pre-clinical evidence for the use of phosphodiesterase-5 inhibitors for treating benign prostatic hyperplasia and lower urinary tract symptoms. *BJU Int* 2006;98: 1259-1263.

14.  Lee C, Kozlowski JM, Grayhack JT: Intrinsic and extrinsic factors controlling benign prostatic growth. *Prostate* 1997;31:131-138.

15.  Behre HM, Bohmeyer J, Nieschlag E: Prostate volume in testosterone-treated and untreated hypogonadal men in comparison to age-matched normal controls. *Clin Endocrinol (Oxf)* 1994;40: 341-349.

16.  Wilson JD: The pathogenesis of benign prostatic hyperplasia. *Am J Med* 1980;68:745-756.

17.  Lee C, Sensibar JA, Dudek SM, et al: Prostatic ductal system in rats: regional variation in morphological and functional activities. *Biol Reprod* 1990;43:1079-1086.

18.  Sensibar JA, Griswold MD, Sylvester SR, et al: Prostatic ductal system in rats: regional variation in localization of an androgen-repressed gene product, sulfated glycoprotein-2. *Endocrinology* 1991;128:2091-2102.

19.  Sherwood ER, Fong CJ, Lee C, et al: Basic fibroblast growth factor: a potential mediator of stromal growth in the human prostate. *Endocrinology* 1992;130:2955-2963.

20.  Stoller ML, Carroll PR: Urology. In: Tierney LM Jr, McPhee SJ, Papadakis MA, eds: *Current Medical Diagnosis and Treatment*, 43rd ed. New York, NY, Lange Medical Books/McGraw-Hill, 2004, p 922.

21.  Grayhack JT, Sensibar JA, Ilio KY: Synergistic action of steroids and spermatocele fluid on in vitro proliferation of prostate stroma. *J Urol* 1998;159:2202-2209.

229

22. Grayhack JT, Kozlowski JM, Lee C: The pathogenesis of benign prostatic hyperplasia: a proposed hypothesis and critical evaluation. *J Urol* 1998;160(6 pt 2):2375-2380.

23. Issa MM, Marshall F: Anatomy of the genitourinary system. In: *Contemporary Diagnosis and Management of Diseases of the Prostate*, 3rd ed. Newtown, PA, Handbooks in Health Care Co., 2005, pp 5-12.

24. Scher HI: Hyperplastic and malignant diseases of the prostate. In: Braunwald E, Fauci AS, Kasper DL, et al, eds: *Harrison's Principles of Internal Medicine*, 15th ed. New York, NY, McGraw-Hill, 2001, pp 608-616.

25. Anderson JB, Roehrborn CG, Schalken JA, et al: The progression of benign prostatic hyperplasia: examining the evidence and determining the risk. *Eur Urol* 2001;39:390-399.

26. Isaacs JT, Coffey DS: Changes in dihydrotestosterone metabolism associated with the development of canine benign prostatic hyperplasia. *Endocrinology* 1981;108:445-453.

27. Roehrborn CG, Boyle P, Bergner D, et al: Serum prostate-specific antigen and prostate volume predict long-term changes in symptoms and flow rate: results of a four-year, randomized trial comparing finasteride versus placebo. PLESS Study Group. *Urology* 1999;54:662-669.

28. Roehrborn CG, Malice M, Cook TJ, et al: Clinical predictors of spontaneous acute urinary retention in men with LUTS and clinical BPH: a comprehensive analysis of the pooled placebo groups of several large clinical trials. *Urology* 2001;58:210-216.

29. Michel MC, Mehlburger L, Bressel HU, et al: Comparison of tamsulosin efficacy in subgroups of patients with lower urinary tract symptoms. *Prostate Cancer Prostatic Dis* 1998;1:332-335.

30. Michel MC, Mehlburger L, Bressel HU, et al: Tamsulosin treatment of 19,365 patients with lower urinary tract symptoms: does co-morbidity alter tolerability? *J Urol* 1998;160(6 pt 1):784-791.

31. Ogiste JS, Cooper K, Kaplan SA: Are stents still a useful therapy for benign prostatic hyperplasia? *Curr Opin Urol* 2003;13:51-57.

32. Carraro JC, Raynaud JP, Koch G, et al: Comparison of phytotherapy (Permixon) with finasteride in the treatment of benign prostate hyperplasia: a randomized international study of 1,098 patients. *Prostate* 1996;29:231-240; discussion 241-242.

33. Grasso M, Montesano A, Buonaguidi A, et al: Comparative effects of alfuzosin versus Serenoa repens in the treatment of symptomatic benign prostatic hyperplasia. *Arch Esp Urol* 1995;48:97-103.

34. Ford ES, Giles WH, Dietz WH: Prevalence of the metabolic syndrome among US adults: findings from the third National Health and Nutrition Examination Survey. *JAMA* 2002;287:356-359.

35. Dahle SE, Chokkalingam AP, Gao YT, et al: Body size and serum levels of insulin and leptin in relation to the risk of benign prostatic hyperplasia. *J Urol* 2002;168:599-604.

36. Joseph MA, Harlow SD, Wei JT, et al: Risk factors for lower urinary tract symptoms in a population-based sample of African-American men. *Am J Epidemiol* 2003;157:906-914.

37. Hammarsten J, Hogstedt B: Clinical, anthropometric, metabolic and insulin profile of men with fast annual growth rates of benign prostatic hyperplasia. *Blood Press* 1999;8:29-36.

38. Hammarsten J, Hogstedt B: Hyperinsulinaemia as a risk factor for developing benign prostatic hyperplasia. *Eur Urol* 2001;39:151-158.

39. Bautista OM, Kusek JW, Nyberg LM, et al: Study design of the Medical Therapy of Prostatic Symptoms (MTOPS) trial. *Control Clin Trials* 2003;24:224-243.

40. McConnell JD, Roehrborn CG, Bautista OM, et al, and The Medical Therapy of Prostatic Symptoms (MTOPS) Research Group: The long-term effect of doxazosin, finasteride, and combination therapy on the clinical progression of benign prostatic hyperplasia. *N Engl J Med* 2003;349:2387-2398.

41. Helfand B, Mouli S, Dedhia R, et al: Management of lower urinary tract symptoms secondary to benign prostatic hyperplasia with open prostatectomy: results of a contemporary series. *J Urol* 2006;176(6 pt 1):2557-2561; discussion 2561.

42. Floratos DL, Kiemeney LA, Rossi C, et al: Long-term followup of randomized transurethral microwave thermotherapy versus transurethral prostatic resection study. *J Urol* 2001;165:1533-1538.

43. Grayhack JT, McVary KT, Kozlowski JM: *Benign Prostatic Hyperplasia*. Philadelphia, PA, Lippincott Williams & Wilkins, 2002, pp 1401-1470.

44. Iversen P, Madsen PO: Short-term cephalosporin prophylaxis in transurethral surgery. *Clin Ther* 1982;5(suppl A):58-66.

45. Practice Guidelines Committee: AUA guideline on the management of benign prostatic hyperplasia (2003). Chapter 1: Diagnosis and treatment recommendations. *J Urol* 2003;170(2 pt 1): 530-547.

46. de la Rosette JJ, Laguna MP, Gravas S, et al: Transurethral microwave thermotherapy: the gold standard for minimally invasive therapies for patients with benign prostatic hyperplasia? *J Endourol* 2003;17:245-251.

47. Hallin A, Berlin T: Transurethral microwave thermotherapy for benign prostatic hyperplasia: clinical outcome after 4 years. *J Urol* 1998;159:459-464.

48. Dahlstrand C, Walden M, Geirsson G, et al: Transurethral microwave thermotherapy versus transurethral resection for symptomatic benign prostatic obstruction: a prospective randomized study with a 2-year follow-up. *Br J Urol* 1995;76:614-618.

49. D'Ancona F C, Francisca EA, Witjes WP, et al: High energy thermotherapy versus transurethral resection in the treatment of benign prostatic hyperplasia: results of a prospective randomized study with 1 year of followup. *J Urol* 1997;158:120-125.

50. Schatzl G, Madersbacher S, Djavan B, et al: Two-year results of transurethral resection of the prostate versus four 'less invasive' treatment options. *Eur Urol* 2000;37:695-701.

51. Perry MJ, Roodhouse A, Gidlow AB, et al: Thermo-expandable intraprostatic stents in bladder outlet obstruction: an 8-year study. *BJU Int* 2002;90:216-223.

52. Madersbacher S, Alivizatos G, Nordling J, et al: EAU 2004 guidelines on assessment, therapy and follow-up of men with lower urinary tract symptoms suggestive of benign prostatic obstruction (BPH guidelines). *Eur Urol* 2004;46:547-554.

53. Muschter R: Conductive heat: hot water-induced thermotherapy for ablation of prostatic tissue. *J Endourol* 2003;17:609-616.

54. Issa MM, Marshall F: Transurethral resection of the prostate and similar procedures. In: *Contemporary Diagnosis and Management of Diseases of the Prostate,* 3rd ed. Newtown, PA, Handbooks in Health Care Co, 2005, pp 100-108.

55. Roehrborn CG: Management. In: *Contemporary Diagnosis and Management of Benign Prostatic Hyperplasia.* Newtown, PA, Handbooks in Health Care Co, 2005, pp 90-187.

56. Hahn RG: Transurethral resection syndrome from extravascular absorption of irrigating fluid. *Scand J Urol Nephrol* 1993;27:387-394.

57. Rassweiler J, Schulze M, Stock C, et al: Bipolar transurethral resection of the prostate—technical modifications and early clinical experience. *Minim Invasive Ther Allied Technol* 2007;16:11-21.

58. Roehrborn CG: Natural history. In: *Contemporary Diagnosis and Management of Benign Prostatic Hyperplasia*. Newtown, PA, Handbooks in Health Care Co, 2005, pp 47-69.

59. Issa MM, Marshall F: Benign prostatic hyperplasia. In: *Contemporary Diagnosis and Management of Diseases of the Prostate*, 3rd ed. Newtown, PA, Handbooks in Health Care Co, 2005, pp 13-47.

60. Chute CG, Panser LA, Girman CJ, et al: The prevalence of prostatism: a population-based survey of urinary symptoms. *J Urol* 1993;150:85-89.

61. Lepor H, Machi G: Comparison of AUA symptom index in unselected males and females between fifty-five and seventy-nine years of age. *Urology* 1993;42:36-40; discussion 40-41.

62. Sanda MG, Beaty TH, Stutzman RE, et al: Genetic susceptibility of benign prostatic hyperplasia. *J Urol* 1994;152:115-119.

63. Sanda MG, Doehring CB, Binkowitz B, et al: Clinical and biological characteristics of familial benign prostatic hyperplasia. *J Urol* 1997;157:876-879.

64. Kristal AR, Arnold KB, Schenk JM, et al: Race/ethnicity, obesity, health related behaviors and the risk of symptomatic benign prostatic hyperplasia: results from the prostate cancer prevention trial. *J Urol* 2007;177:1395-1400.

65. Zucchetto A, Tavani A, Dal Maso L, et al: History of weight and obesity through life and risk of benign prostatic hyperplasia. *Int J Obes (Lond)* 2005;29:798-803.

66. Glynn RJ, Campion EW, Bouchard GR, et al: The development of benign prostatic hyperplasia among volunteers in the Normative Aging Study. *Am J Epidemiol* 1985;121:78-90.

67. Girman CJ, Panser LA, Chute CG, et al: Natural history of prostatism: urinary flow rates in a community-based study. *J Urol* 1993;150:887-892.

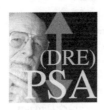

# Index

# U

# NOTES

# NOTES

# NOTES

# NOTES

# NOTES